Peptides in Nanotechnology

Among the various nanomaterials, peptides have emerged as a promising tool due to their unique properties such as high specificity, biocompatibility, and low toxicity. This book provides a comprehensive overview of the field of peptide-based nanomaterials, from their synthesis to their applications. It covers the latest advancements in peptide nanotechnology and provides detailed insights into various aspects of peptide-based nanomaterials, including their properties, synthesis, characterization, and potential applications in various biomedical fields.

Features:

- Provides up-to-date detailed descriptions of various peptide-based nanostructures and their formation.
- Covers a wide range of topics related to peptides in nanotechnology including their synthesis and characterization.
- Includes the latest research and developments in the field of peptides in nanotechnology.
- Contains recent applications in drug delivery, tissue engineering, imaging and diagnostics, and targeted cancer therapy.
- Reviews peptide-nanoparticle conjugates (PNCs).

This book is aimed at graduate students and researchers in peptide synthesis, biomedical engineering, and drug development and delivery.

Peptides in Nanotechnology

Laksiri Weerasinghe and
Saranya Selvaraj

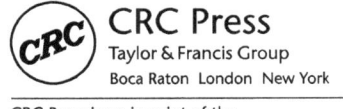
CRC Press
Taylor & Francis Group
Boca Raton London New York

CRC Press is an imprint of the
Taylor & Francis Group, an **informa** business

Designed cover image: Shutterstock

First edition published 2025
by CRC Press
2385 NW Executive Center Drive, Suite 320, Boca Raton FL 33431

and by CRC Press
4 Park Square, Milton Park, Abingdon, Oxon, OX14 4RN

CRC Press is an imprint of Taylor & Francis Group, LLC

© 2025 Laksiri Weerasinghe and Saranya Selvaraj

Reasonable efforts have been made to publish reliable data and information, but the author and publisher cannot assume responsibility for the validity of all materials or the consequences of their use. The authors and publishers have attempted to trace the copyright holders of all material reproduced in this publication and apologize to copyright holders if permission to publish in this form has not been obtained. If any copyright material has not been acknowledged please write and let us know so we may rectify in any future reprint.

Except as permitted under U.S. Copyright Law, no part of this book may be reprinted, reproduced, transmitted, or utilized in any form by any electronic, mechanical, or other means, now known or hereafter invented, including photocopying, microfilming, and recording, or in any information storage or retrieval system, without written permission from the publishers.

For permission to photocopy or use material electronically from this work, access www.copyright.com or contact the Copyright Clearance Center, Inc. (CCC), 222 Rosewood Drive, Danvers, MA 01923, 978-750-8400. For works that are not available on CCC please contact mpkbookspermissions@tandf.co.uk

Trademark notice: Product or corporate names may be trademarks or registered trademarks and are used only for identification and explanation without intent to infringe.

ISBN: 9781032661971 (hbk)
ISBN: 9781041020837 (pbk)
ISBN: 9781003617686 (ebk)

DOI: 10.1201/9781003617686

Typeset in Times
by codeMantra

Contents

Preface ix
Acknowledgments xi
Author biographies xiii

Chapter 1 Introduction to peptides in nanotechnology 1

    1.1 Introduction to peptides 1
    1.2 Peptides and nanotechnology 2
    1.3 Importance of peptides in nanotechnology 3
    1.4 Historical background of peptides in nanotechnology 4
    1.5 Classification of peptides 6
    1.6 Properties of peptides in nanotechnology 7
    1.7 Advantages and challenges of using peptides in nanotechnology 8
        1.7.1 Advantages of using peptides in nanotechnology ... 8
        1.7.2 Challenges of using peptides in nanotechnology 9
    1.8 Applications of peptides in nanotechnology 10
        1.8.1 Peptide-based drug delivery systems 10
        1.8.2 Peptide-based imaging agents 10
        1.8.3 Peptide-based tissue engineering and regenerative medicine 10
        1.8.4 Peptide-based vaccines 10
        1.8.5 Peptide-based nanomaterials 10
    1.9 Prospects of peptides in nanotechnology 11
    1.10 Practice questions 12

Chapter 2 Synthesis and characterization of peptides 15

    2.1 Peptide and chemical synthesis 15
    2.2 Biological synthesis 15
    2.3 Ribosomal synthesis 17
    2.4 Non-ribosomal synthesis 18
    2.5 Chemical synthesis of peptides 18
        2.5.1 Solid-Phase Peptide Synthesis 19
        2.5.2 Coupling reaction 23
        2.5.3 Deprotection 27
        2.5.4 New trends in SPPS 28
        2.5.5 Limitations of SPPS 30
        2.5.6 Liquid/Solution-Phase Peptide Synthesis 31

	2.6	Hybrid peptide synthesis 34
		2.6.1 Strategies for hybrid peptide synthesis..................34
		2.6.2 Challenges in hybrid peptide synthesis 36
		2.6.3 Recent advances in hybrid peptide synthesis 37
	2.7	Purification and characterization of peptides.....................38
	2.8	Mass spectrometry and NMR spectroscopy 40
		2.8.1 Mass Spectrometry..40
		2.8.2 NMR Spectroscopy 41
	2.9	Other methods for peptide characterization 41
	2.10	Recent advances in peptide synthesis and characterization 42
		2.10.1 Peptide synthesis 42
		2.10.2 Peptide characterization 43
	2.11	Practical questions..43

Chapter 3 Peptide-based nanostructures..52

	3.1	Introduction to peptide-based nanostructures 52
	3.2	Peptide self-assembly 53
	3.3	Peptide amphiphilic...54
	3.4	Peptide-based NPs...55
	3.5	Peptide-based hydrogels 56
	3.6	Peptide nanotubes and nanorods 57
		3.6.1 Preparation of nanotubes..57
		3.6.2 Difference between peptide nanotubes and nanorods 59
	3.7	Peptide-based nanocomposites..62
	3.8	Characterization of peptide-based nanostructures.............62
	3.9	Applications of peptide-based nanostructures 63
	3.10	Future prospects of peptide-based nanostructures............64
	3.11	Practical questions...65

Chapter 4 Peptides for drug delivery with nanomaterials 70

	4.1	Introduction to peptide-based nano delivery systems 70
	4.2	Peptide-based nanocarriers for drug delivery 74
	4.3	Application peptide-mediated drug delivery systems 75
	4.4	CPPs for drug delivery 77
		4.4.1 Mechanisms of CPP 78
	4.5	Targeted drug delivery using peptides...............................79
	4.6	Stimuli-responsive peptides...82
	4.7	AMPs and anticancer peptides...84
	4.8	Challenges and prospects of peptide-based drug delivery ...85

Chapter 5 Applications of peptide-conjugated nanomaterials......................95

	5.1	General applications of peptide-conjugated nanomaterials 95

	5.2	Introduction to peptide-based sensors and biosensors 95
		5.2.1 Peptide-based biosensors for disease diagnosis, environmental monitoring, and food quality control 99
	5.3	Introduction to peptide-based tissue engineering and regenerative medicine 101
		5.3.1 Peptide-based biomaterial scaffolds and hydrogels for tissue engineering 104
	5.4	Introduction to peptide-based imaging and diagnostic 106
		5.4.1 Peptide-based imaging agents and probes for disease diagnosis 106
		5.4.2 Peptide-based probes for imaging of biological processes 109
	5.5	Introduction to peptide-based targeting of cancer cells 111
		5.5.1 Peptide-conjugated chemotherapeutic and immunotherapy agents 112
	5.6	Peptide-based vaccines 113
		5.6.1 Peptide-based vaccines for infectious diseases, cancer, allergies, and autoimmune diseases 113
		5.6.2 Peptide-conjugated chemotherapeutic and immunotherapy agents 115
	5.7	Practical questions 117

Chapter 6 Future directions and challenges in peptide nanotechnology 124

	6.1	Introduction 124
	6.2	Emerging trends in peptide nanotechnology 125
	6.3	Challenges in peptide synthesis and characterization 127
	6.4	Challenges in peptide-based nanomaterials 129
	6.5	Regulatory challenges in peptide-based therapeutics 130
	6.6	Ethical and social challenges in peptide nanotechnology 131
	6.7	Future directions and opportunities in peptide nanotechnology 132
	6.8	Conclusions and final thoughts of peptides in nanotechnology 134
	6.9	Practical questions 135

Index 137

Preface

Peptides are short chains of amino acids and the building blocks of life, and they play pivotal roles in both biology and chemistry fields. Their versatility extends far beyond their biological functions, as scientists have harnessed the power of peptides to produce resourceful nanotechnological applications. Nanotechnology, the science and engineering of manipulating matter at the nanometer scale, has been a driving force behind countless breakthroughs in various scientific and industrial domains. This book incorporates the intriguing convergence of peptides in nanotechnology, exploring the synthesis, manipulation, and transformative potential of peptide-based nanostructures and their applications.

As you read through the pages of this book, we will research the elegance of peptide design, the precision of nanoscale assembly, and the countless applications that range from targeted drug delivery to the development of advanced biomaterials. This book is not a mere collection of facts and figures; instead, it is an invitation to embark on a journey of the elegance of scientific theories at the start but has been invented for various applications. This book also speaks on the synthesis, purification, characterization, and nanostructures incorporated with peptides while exploring several applications including drugs based on peptides and nanotechnology.

This book is intended not only for the scientist and researcher but also for the curious minds eager to grasp the marvels of this emerging field, especially students in both chemistry and biology fields. Whether you are a student, a teacher, a scientist, an entrepreneur, or simply someone with an insatiable curiosity about the world around you, there is something here for you.

We expect that this book will function as a comprehensive reference guide, providing a detailed examination of how peptides play a major role in nanotechnology while spotlighting the fascinating recent discoveries in this field.

– **Laksiri Weerasinghe**

Acknowledgments

As we reflect on the completion of this book on *Peptide in Nanotechnology*, I am deeply grateful to all those who have played a part in its creation. Writing a book is a journey that involves countless hours of research, writing, and editing. It is also a collaborative effort that relies on the support and contributions of numerous individuals and organizations.

We extend our appreciation to my colleagues and fellow researchers in the field of nanotechnology and biotechnology. Your insights, discussions, and collaboration have enriched my knowledge and expanded the scope of this book.

We would like to acknowledge the countless scientists, researchers, and innovators who have contributed to the advancement of peptide nanotechnology field. Your pioneering work has paved the way for the discoveries and applications discussed in this book.

Our heartfelt thanks go to our families for their unwavering support and understanding during the demanding process of writing and research. Your belief in my work has been a constant source of motivation.

We are also grateful to the team at CRC Press for their professionalism, expertise, and dedication to bringing this book to fruition. Your editorial and production efforts have transformed my manuscript into a polished and accessible publication.

Lastly, we want to express my gratitude to the readers and enthusiasts of science and technology who will embark on this intellectual journey with me. Your curiosity and interest in the world of peptide nanotechnology are what drive the dissemination of knowledge and the pursuit of innovation.

This book would not have been possible without the collective efforts of all those mentioned and the countless others who have contributed in various ways. It is a testament to the collaborative spirit of the scientific community and the enduring quest for knowledge.

– **Laksiri Weerasinghe and Saranya Selvaraj**

Author biographies

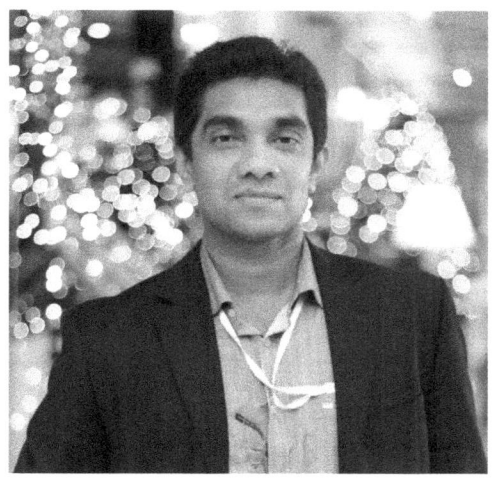

Laksiri Weerasinghe is currently a senior lecturer, Department of Chemistry, Faculty of Applied Sciences, University of Sri Jayewardenepura (USJP). He obtained his BSc Honors degree in Chemistry from the University of Colombo, Sri Lanka. Then he earned his doctoral degree from Washington State University, USA, under the guidance of Prof. Phill Garner in the field of synthetic organic chemistry. He completed his postdoctoral studies at the University of Montreal, Canada, in 2013–2014 under the guidance of Prof. Stephence Hannesian and the second postdoctoral training at Washington State University in 2014–2015 under the guidance of Prof. Ming Xian.

After returning to Sri Lanka, he worked as a senior research scientist in Sri Lanka Institute of Nanotechnology (SLINTEC) for five years before joining the faculty at USJP. At SLINTEC, he was the leading scientist of synthetic organic and pharmaceutical division. With a strategic research grant from the Ministry of Research and Development, he established the first bioorganic laboratory at SLINTEC with state-of-the-art facilities for peptide synthesis. His independent research interests are mainly addressing the challenges in drug discovery and drug delivery using organic synthesis and nanotechnology. In addition to small molecular synthesis, he also works on antimicrobial peptides, realizing their potential in plant science and agriculture.

With his independent research contributions, he has more than 25 research papers in peer-reviewed journals, two books, one book chapter, and many conference proceedings. He received the President's Award for Scientific Research in 2018 and Support Scheme for Supervision of Research Degrees (SUSRED) award in 2023.

He has been a member of the council of the Institute of Chemistry Ceylon since 2022 and the chairperson of All Island Interschool Chemistry Quiz Committee.

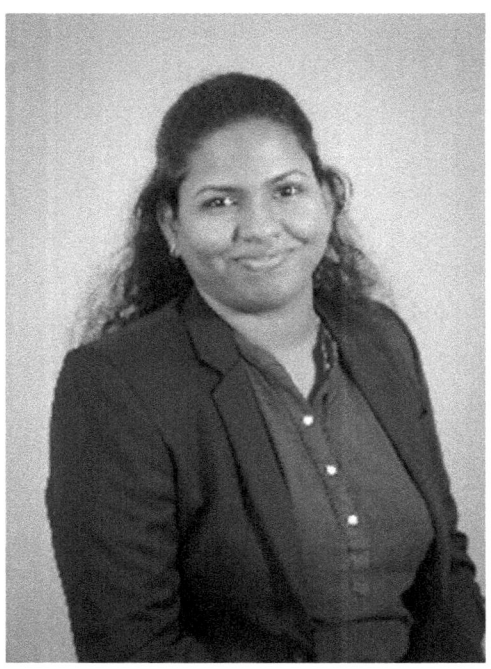

Saranya Selvaraj began her academic journey with a Bachelor of Science in Biotechnology, Microbiology, and Biochemistry from the University of Mysore, India. Pursuing her passion for biotechnology, she obtained her Master of Science in the same field from the University of Peradeniya, Sri Lanka, while conducting her research at the Biotechnology Unit, Industrial Technology Institute (ITI), Sri Lanka. Her education laid a strong foundation for her to explore and excel in the scientific arena. Currently, she is pursuing an MPhil in Chemistry at the University of Sri Jayewardenepura, Sri Lanka. In addition to her studies, she serves as a graduate research assistant at the Department of Chemistry, Faculty of Applied Science, at the same university. She is also affiliated with the Centre for Scientific Computing and Advanced Drug Discovery as well as the Idea Lab within the Department of Zoology and Environmental Science at the University of Colombo. Her research specializes in Peptide Chemistry, Material Science, and Nanotechnology, focusing on the synthesis, characterization, and manipulation of bioactive compounds at the nanoscale for therapeutic applications. She has made significant contributions through her independent research, including the publication of a few research papers and literature reviews in peer-reviewed journals, and numerous conference presentations. Saranya is currently a Visiting Lecturer at the European City Campus, Sri Lanka, and a Volunteer with ReachSci, a society offering training programs to help researchers develop skills and tackle global challenges. She combines her expertise with a passion for teaching, and mentoring students to excel in research and STEM fields.

1 Introduction to peptides in nanotechnology

1.1 INTRODUCTION TO PEPTIDES

Short sequences of amino acid residues connected by amide linkages are referred to as peptides.[1] Traditionally, peptides with fewer than 20 amino acids are referred to as oligopeptides, and those with between 20 and 100 amino acids are referred to as polypeptides. Structurally (Figure 1.1), peptides are arranged in an array of structural forms including linear, cyclic, and depsipeptides. Modified peptides with various nonpeptide moieties, such as phosphoryl groups or carbohydrates (phosphopeptides or glycopeptides), polyketides, or terpenoids, are also found in nature.[2]

Besides their unique biological activities, peptides have gained a great deal of interest recently due to their unique features such as biocompatibility, stability, and specificity. With their potential use in biosensing, tissue engineering, and drug delivery, peptide-based nanostructures have gained a great deal of interest recently in the realm of nanotechnology.[3] However, understanding the fundamentals of peptides including the synthesis and characterization is key to the expansion of their application in nanotechnology.

The principles of peptide synthesis involve the sequential joining of amino acids to create peptide chains.[4] Primarily, peptide synthesis can be done using

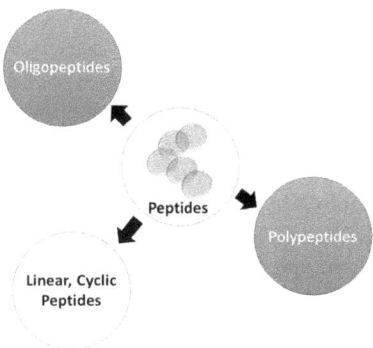

FIGURE 1.1 Different structure of peptides.

solid-phase peptide synthesis (SPPS), liquid-phase peptide synthesis, and native chemical ligation. Currently, the most common method is SPPS, in which the process of creating peptides by joining the initial amino acid to a solid support, adding subsequent amino acids one by one, and finally splitting the peptide from the solid support.[5] Protecting groups also play a critical role by ensuring the chemo-selective in peptide synthesis.[6] More details including manual, automated, and microwave-assisted peptide synthesizers and their advantages and disadvantages are discussed in detail in Chapter 2.

1.2 PEPTIDES AND NANOTECHNOLOGY

Peptides and nanotechnology are two distinct fields that have emerged as crucial tools in the biomedical sciences in recent years. Hence, a basic understanding of each field could be useful for future scientists and science contributors in peptides and nanotechnology.

Engineering and manipulating materials on a nanoscale is the field of nanotechnology (generally between the scale of 1 and 100 nm).[7] Nanomaterials with a diameter in the range of 1–100 nm, for instance, however one dimension outside the nanoscale, include nanorods, nanowires, and nanofibers. A single material or a combination of materials can be used to create nanostructured materials, which are nanomaterials with one dimension in the nanoscale range (less than 100 nm). Hence, nanostructured materials are made of interconnected nanoscale pieces.[8] Simple materials (such as metal, carbon, and polymers) may be employed to create nanoparticles and nanostructured structures,[9] composites (e.g., polymer-metal, silica-metal, graphene-metal), or in core-shell forms. Nanotechnology has enabled the development of materials and devices with unique properties and uses including customized medication delivery, bioimaging, and biosensors.

Peptides have emerged as a versatile tool in nanotechnology due to their facility to self-assembling into various nanostructures such as nanotubes, nanofibers, and nanoparticles. These peptide-based nanostructures have unique properties that make them ideal for various applications, such as drug delivery, imaging, and tissue engineering.[10] Additionally, peptides can be used to functionalize the surfaces of nanoparticles to improve their stability, targeting, and cellular uptake.[11] Nanotechnology has also revolutionized the field of peptide synthesis and characterization. Advanced analytical techniques such as mass spectrometry, nuclear magnetic resonance (NMR), and X-ray crystallography have also enabled researchers to determine the structures and properties of peptides at the atomic level. Nanoparticles and nanomaterials have also been used to improve the efficiency of peptide synthesis and purification.[12]

Peptides and nanotechnology are two distinct fields that have become increasingly intertwined in recent years. Peptide-based nanostructures have emerged as new avenues for medication delivery, imaging, and tissue engineering. Understanding the fundamental characteristics of these two fields is essential for advancing biomedical research and developing innovative technologies.

Introduction to peptides in nanotechnology

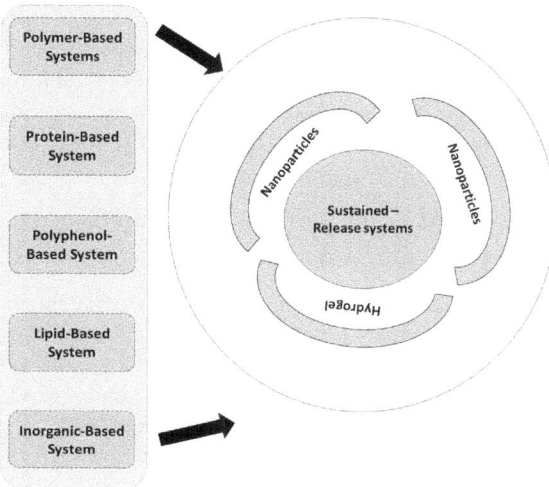

FIGURE 1.2 Sustainable application of peptide drugs, recreated with content from Sustained Release Systems for Delivery of Therapeutic Peptide/Protein. "Copyright 2001 ACS Publication".

1.3 IMPORTANCE OF PEPTIDES IN NANOTECHNOLOGY

Peptides are regarded as one of the essential biomaterials in nanotechnology because of their distinctive chemical and physical properties. An overview of the significance of peptides in nanotechnology will be given in this section (Figure 1.2).

Building blocks called peptides are used to create and develop nanomaterials with certain features. The incorporation of peptides into nanomaterials imparts a range of desirable features such as improved stability, biocompatibility, and targeting abilities. Peptide-based nanomaterials have been used in a variety of applications, including tissue engineering, medication delivery, and biosensors.[13] Peptide-based drug delivery systems can target specific cells or tissues, thus reducing off-target effects and improving therapeutic efficacy.[14] For example, targeting cancer cells has been done with peptide-conjugated nanoparticles, resulting in improved drug delivery and enhanced anticancer activity.[15]

Another application of peptides has been extensively used as molecular probes for imaging and sensing applications in nanotechnology. The unique sequence and structure of peptides enable their use as molecular probes for specific biomolecules, including proteins, nucleic acids, and small molecules.[16] Peptide-based probes have been used in various imaging techniques such as magnetic resonance imaging (MRI), computed tomography (CT), and positron emission tomography (PET).[14]

Due to their capacity to encourage cell adhesion, proliferation, and differentiation, peptides have found widespread application in tissue engineering and regenerative medicine. Peptide-based scaffolds have been used to mimic the extracellular matrix (ECM) and guide tissue regeneration.[17] Additionally, peptide-based growth factors have been used to enhance tissue repair and regeneration.

Due to their inherent ability to bind specifically to target molecules, peptide probes have also been useful in the development of nano-biosensors. Many analytes, including proteins, nucleic acids, and small-sized molecules, have been detected by employing peptide-based biosensors. Moreover, peptide-based biosensors are frequently employed to find various pathogenic and cancer biomarkers.[18]

1.4 HISTORICAL BACKGROUND OF PEPTIDES IN NANOTECHNOLOGY

Peptides have been incorporated into nanotechnology since the early 1990s. The potential of peptides as building blocks for nanostructures was first recognized by Ghadiri and coworkers.[19] Since then, various investigations into the usage of peptides in nanotechnology have been performed, and many peptide-based nanomaterials have been developed for a wide range of biomedical applications.

Despite all the excitement surrounding it in recent years for the nanotechnology field, there are pieces of evidence to take it back to the Romans, who imitated the coloration of butterfly wings about 1600 years ago. The glass mug known as the Lycurgus cup in the British Museum contains nanoparticles of gold and silver which appear jade green in ambient light and a striking crimson color when a powerful light shines through it. Nanoparticles in the sky are what give sunsets their red and yellow hues, while carbon nanoparticles are used in the production of vehicle tires.[20] Over 2000 years ago, Indian artisans and craftspeople employed nanotechnology to create weapons and durable cave paintings, and research has revealed the presence of carbon nanoparticles in Tipu Sultan's famous sword and the Ajanta paintings, two of the country's oldest cave paintings.[21]

In the early days, peptide-based nanomaterials were mainly used for drug delivery applications. One of the earliest examples was the development of liposomes decked with cyclic RGD peptides (arginine–glycine–aspartic peptides) for targeted carriers of anticancer drugs. Another early example was the development of nanoparticles composed of a block copolymer and a peptide that targeted $\alpha v\beta 3$ integrin receptors for imaging and drug delivery applications.[22] Peptide-based nanomaterials have now been created for a variety of applications as the area has rapidly grown, including cancer therapy, tissue engineering, biosensors, and imaging. The development of various peptide-drug conjugates was facilitated through the application of peptides to enhance the stability and solubility of poorly soluble medicines.

The use of peptides in nanotechnology has also been driven by advances in peptide synthesis techniques. SPPS, which was first presented in the 1960s, has revolutionized the field of peptide chemistry and has made it possible to synthesize peptides with a high degree of purity and accuracy. SPPS has also enabled the synthesis of complex peptides, including cyclic peptides and peptide-based macrocycles, which have been appealing for use in nanotechnology applications because of their distinctive qualities.

The historical background of peptides in nanotechnology highlighting the rich history of peptide-based materials and their contributions to the development of nanotechnology has been summarized in Table 1.1. The field has rapidly advanced, and currently, peptides have become essential building blocks for the production of different nanomaterials for use in biomedical fields.

TABLE 1.1
The historical background of peptide development

Year	Historical importance	References
1925	Richard Zsigmondy, a chemistry Nobel Prize winner from 1925, was the first to propose the idea of a "nanometer." He was the initial person to employ a microscope to determine the size of particles like gold colloids, and he was the one who originally used the term "nanometer" to characterize the particle size.	23
1965	Richard Feynman won the physics Nobel Prize in 1965. "There's Plenty of Space at the Bottom," a talk he gave at the 1959 American Physical Society meeting at Caltech. He proposed the concept of atomic-level manipulation of matter.	24
1963	Synthesis of the peptide using Solid phase peptide synthesis	25
1970	The term "nanotechnology" was first used to refer to semiconductor operations that transpired at a distance of around a nanometer from a Japanese scientist named Norio Taniguchi. He argued that the processing, separation, consolidation, and deformation of materials by one atom or one molecule included nanotechnology.	23
1983	The first synthesis of a peptide with a metal-binding domain was reported, which opened up new possibilities for using peptides in materials science	26
1902	Richard Zsigmondy used an ultramicroscope to conduct the first observations and measurements of the sizes of nanoparticles.	27
1907	Paul Ehrlich conducted the compounds with original structures designed to specifically target diseases and used for the first time the expression of "magic bullets."	28
1990s	Researchers began to explore the use of peptides for self-assembly into nanostructures, leading to the development of peptide-based nanomaterials.	29
1991	Sumio Iijima discovered carbon nanotubes	30
2002	It was reported that peptides were used for the first time as blueprints for the synthesis of nanoparticles, enabling the production of very homogenous nanoparticles with precise sizes and shapes.	31
2006	Peptide-based hydrogels were developed, which could be used for tissue regeneration and medication delivery	32
2010	Peptide-based nanomaterials were shown to have antimicrobial properties, opening up new possibilities for their use in the development of new antibiotics.	31
2015	Researchers developed a peptide-based coating for nanoparticles that improved their stability and biocompatibility	33
2018	A new type of peptide-based nanomaterials called "peptide nucleic acids" (PNAs) was developed for use in gene therapy.	34

1.5 CLASSIFICATION OF PEPTIDES

Peptides are classified based on their function, sequence, structure, and size. In nanotechnology, peptides have been classified based on the capacity of these molecules to self-assemble into nanoscale structures, as well as their numerous possible application fields such as drug carrier, tissue engineering, and biosensing.[35] An outline will be provided in this section regarding the different classifications of peptides in nanotechnology.

Self-assembling peptides (SAPs) are peptides that have the potential to dynamically form organized nanostructure levels.[36] These peptides can also produce an extensive range of nanostructures, such as nanofibers, nanotubes, nanorods, and nanoparticles. With their ability to mimic the self-assembly behavior of proteins, SAPs are widely applicable in several fields including medication carrying, tissue engineering, and biosensing.

Self-assembly, a procedure that doesn't use any energy, and self-organization, which does an energy-consuming activity, are essentially what comprise the so-called bottom-up assembly. Contrarily, nanoarchitectonics covers fabrication methods including top-down nanofabrication and manipulation more thoroughly. It is claimed that the blending of bottom-up and top-down processes is crucial for the procedure of functional material systems.[37] Certain methods decrease bulk materials to create nanostructures. By using breaking, cutting, or etching techniques, such as mass or film machining, surface machining, and mold machining with lithography, "top-down" manufacturing is achieved. Whereas mold machining uses soft lithography, bulk machining employs photolithography, which applies the etching process.[38] Micro-electro-mechanical system lithography, X-ray lithography, and electron beam lithography are further methods. However, due to their limits in producing nanostructures smaller than 100 nm, photolithography and similar techniques are inapplicable for smaller nanostructures.[39]

SAPs that can create a three-dimensional network of nanofibers are used to create peptide-based hydrogels. These hydrogels have a high-water content and are potentially applied in various biomedical applications, such as wound healing, drug delivery, and tissue engineering. Hydrogels with peptides have the advantage of being biocompatible, biodegradable, and easy to synthesize.[40]

Cell-penetrating peptides (CPPs) are peptides that are minimal enough to enter cells through the cell membrane without causing cell damage. CPPs are applied in drug delivery and gene therapy because they deliver therapeutic molecules to the interior of the cell.[41] CPPs are adaptable to different functional groups, such as fluorescent dyes or targeting moieties, to improve their specificity and efficacy.

Peptide-based nanoparticles are formed from SAPs that can form nanoscale particles. There is a large surface area-to-volume ratio in these nanoparticles, which makes them ideal for use for imaging and medication delivery. These particles are used to increase the accuracy and effectiveness while they can befunctionalized with targeted molecules or imaging agents.

Antimicrobial peptides (AMPs) are peptides with the capacity to eradicate or stop the development of microorganisms, including bacteria, viruses, and fungi.

AMPs have been utilized for a variety of applications, including wound healing, food preservation, and drug discovery. AMPs can be synthesized with modifications to improve their stability and efficacy.[42]

1.6 PROPERTIES OF PEPTIDES IN NANOTECHNOLOGY

Peptides are small biological molecules with unique chemical and physical materials that have features that render them desirable for usage in different fields, including nanotechnology. In this chapter, we will discuss the properties of peptides that make them useful in nanotechnology applications (Figure 1.3).

Peptides have several chemical properties that make them useful in nanotechnology. One of the most important is their ability to form strong, specific interactions with other molecules. This is caused by the presence of functional groups in the peptide chain's amino acid residues. For example, the amino group ($-NH_2$) and a carboxyl group ($-COOH$) on each end of the peptide can form hydrogen bonds with other molecules, allowing peptides to link with specific targets with high affinity and preciseness.[43] Additionally, some amino acids have unique chemical properties. The sulfur-containing amino acid cysteine can form disulfide bonds with other cysteine residues to create stable three-dimensional structures.[44]

Peptides also have several physical properties that make them useful in nanotechnology. Their size represents one of their most crucial characteristics. Peptides are typically much smaller than proteins, from a few hundred to several thousand molecular weight daltons. This small size makes them ideal for use in nanoscale applications, where precise control over size and shape is critical. Another important physical property of peptides is their conformational flexibility. Peptides can adopt a wide range of conformations, including helical,

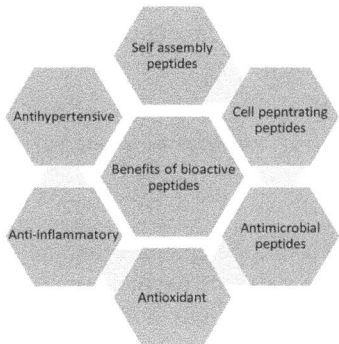

FIGURE 1.3 Different benefits of bioactive peptides have been shown in the diagram Fig 1.3. The functional benefits and classifications of the peptides are considerably altered according to the sources of the peptides. The sources of peptides are diverse and primarily based on the plants and animals, including soy, cereals (such as wheat, barley, rice, rye, oat, millet, sorghum, and corn), and olives; while animals products have examples of different sources milk, egg, meat, and even marine animals.[53]

beta-sheet, and random coil structures. This flexibility allows peptides to fold into specific three-dimensional shapes and interact with other molecules in a variety of ways. Finally, peptides have also excellent biocompatibility and biodegradability, which make them ideal for use in biomedical applications. They can be synthesized from natural amino acids or modified amino acids to enhance their properties and can be easily degraded by natural processes in the body.[45]

1.7 ADVANTAGES AND CHALLENGES OF USING PEPTIDES IN NANOTECHNOLOGY

According to the concept of nano architectonics, useful materials can be designed utilizing nanoscale units that are dependent on the principles of nanotechnology. Functional materials can be produced utilizing nano architectonics methods by combining and picking from a variety of unit processes, such as molecular synthesis, atom/molecule manipulation, self-assembly/self-organization, field-applied assembly, micro-fabrication, and bio-related processes.[46]

Nanoarchitectonics techniques are relevant to a high spectrum of objectives, from physical devices to biomedical applications, due to the widespread use of these processes irrespective of the content or objective. Nanotechnology and nanoarchitecture are both vast, all-encompassing concepts. There is a lot of overlap and shared problems as a result. Both nanotechnology and nano architectonics are responsible for some functional nanostructures' creation and functional outcomes. Yet, their fundamental characteristics and definitions diverge: nanoarchitecture is a process for creating materials and systems from nanoscale things, while nanotechnology is a technology for manipulating nanoscale items.[47]

Peptides have shown great potential in various fields of nanotechnology because of having distinctive qualities like biocompatibility, stability, and functionality. In this section, we will discuss the advantages and limitations of utilizing peptides in nanotechnology.

1.7.1 Advantages of Using Peptides in Nanotechnology

1.7.1.1 Biocompatibility
Peptides are naturally occurring compounds that are biocompatible and biodegradable, therefore a prime prospect for biomedical applications. They do not cause any immune response or toxicity and can be easily metabolized by the body.[48]

1.7.1.2 Diversity
Peptides are highly diverse in their sequences, structures, and functions, providing a wide range of possibilities for their use in nanotechnology. They can be easily synthesized and modified, enabling the development of diverse functional peptide-based nanostructures.

Introduction to peptides in nanotechnology

1.7.1.3 Specificity

Peptides can specifically interact with their target molecules or cells, which is crucial for targeted drug delivery and imaging. Peptides can be made to target certain biomolecules or cell surface receptors, allowing for the targeted delivery of medicines or imaging tools to the desired site.[48]

1.7.1.4 Stability

Peptides are ideal for usage in a variety of environments due to their stability in a wide range of pH and temperature settings in various environments. Additionally, they can be engineered to be resistant to proteolytic degradation, enhancing their stability and half-life *in vivo*.[48]

1.7.2 CHALLENGES OF USING PEPTIDES IN NANOTECHNOLOGY

1.7.2.1 Synthesis

Peptide synthesis can be complicated and time-constraining, especially for longer peptides. Additionally, the low overall yield of the peptide synthesis can limit the amount of peptides that can be produced.

1.7.2.2 Characterization

Peptide characterization can be complex and requires various analytical techniques such as mass spectrometry, NMR spectroscopy, and High-performance liquid chromatography (HPLC). These techniques may be expensive and time-consuming and require specialized training.[49]

1.7.2.3 Stability

While peptides are generally stable, they can be susceptible to degradation by proteases, which can limit their use *in vivo*. Strategies to enhance peptide stability, such as chemical modification, can also introduce new challenges such as toxicity and reduced bioactivity. While the specificity of peptides is a major advantage, it can also be a challenge. Peptides may not bind specifically to their intended target or may bind to other off-target molecules, leading to unintended effects.[48]

1.7.2.4 Specificity

While the specificity of peptides is a major advantage, it can also be challenging. Peptides may not bind specifically to their intended target or may bind to other off-target molecules, leading to unintended effects.

In conclusion, peptides offer numerous advantages for use in nanotechnology, such as biocompatibility, diversity, specificity, and stability. However, there are difficulties with their utilization, including synthesis, characterization, stability, and specificity. While creating peptide-based nanostructures for different purposes, it's crucial to properly take into account these benefits and difficulties.

1.8 APPLICATIONS OF PEPTIDES IN NANOTECHNOLOGY

Peptides have gained significant attention in nanotechnology. In this section, we will discuss the different applications of peptides in nanotechnology.

1.8.1 Peptide-based drug delivery systems

Peptides have been used as drugdelivery vehicles due to their ability to target specific cells or tissues. Systems for targeted medicine delivery based on peptides have been created, including cancer therapy, by conjugating drugs with peptides that recognize cancer-specific markers.

Peptide-based biosensors have been developed for the detection of biomolecules and pathogens. Peptides can act as receptors or recognition elements in biosensors, enabling the detection of specific molecules with high sensitivity and selectivity.[50]

1.8.2 Peptide-based imaging agents

Peptides have been used as imaging agents for various imaging techniques, including MRI and PET. Peptide-based imaging agents can target specific cells or tissues, permitting the visualization of biological processes *in vivo*.

1.8.3 Peptide-based tissue engineering and regenerative medicine

Peptides have been used in tissue engineering and regenerative medicine for the development of scaffolds and matrices that mimic the ECM. Moreover, peptides can promote cell differentiation and proliferation, resulting in tissue regeneration.[51]

1.8.4 Peptide-based vaccines

Peptide-based vaccines have been developed for the inhibition and treatment of various diseases, including cancer and infectious diseases. Peptides can stimulate the immune system to produce antibodies against specific antigens.[52]

1.8.5 Peptide-based nanomaterials

Peptides have been used in the synthesis of nanomaterials, including nanoparticles and nanotubes. Peptide-based nanomaterials have unique properties, such as biocompatibility, stability, and self-assembly, that make them suitable for various applications.

1.9 PROSPECTS OF PEPTIDES IN NANOTECHNOLOGY

Peptides have emerged as versatile building blocks in several implications of nanotechnology because they have special physicochemical properties and high biocompatibility. In the last few generations, peptide technology has advanced tremendously with synthesis and characterization, which has led to the development of various peptide-based nanomaterials. These materials possess several desirable properties such as biocompatibility, biodegradability, and the ability to self-assemble, making them ideal for presentations such as drug delivery, tissue engineering, and biosensing.

The growing interest in creating peptide-based nanomaterials has been observed recently with advanced functionalities such as stimuli-responsive behavior, targeting specificity, and controlled release. The ability to incorporate functional moieties into peptides has opened a new avenue for the development of smart nanomaterials that can respond to various external stimuli such as pH, temperature, and light.

One of the most promising applications of peptides in nanotechnology is in the field of drug delivery. Peptide-based drug delivery systems have the potential to improve the therapeutic index of drugs by enhancing their solubility, stability, and bioavailability. Furthermore, peptide-based systems can target specific cells or tissues, limiting the side effects of medication while improving their efficacy.

Peptides also hold great promise in tissue engineering and regenerative medicine. Peptide-based scaffolds can provide a favorable microenvironment for cell growth and tissue regeneration. They can also promote cell adhesion, migration, and differentiation, which are essential for tissue engineering.

Another exciting area of research in peptide nanotechnology is the development of peptide-based biosensors. Such biosensors are capable of detecting a variety of analytes, such as proteins, nucleic acids, and small molecules, with high specificity and sensitivity. Peptide-based biosensors are suitable for a range of uses, such as disease diagnosis, environmental monitoring, and food safety.

Despite the significant advances made in peptide nanotechnology, several challenges remain. One of the main challenges is the lack of robust and scalable methods for peptide synthesis and characterization. Furthermore, the development of peptide-based nanomaterials with advanced knowing the physicochemical characteristics of peptides is critical to comprehending functions, which can be challenging.

Therefore, peptides have shown possibilities for several nanotechnological submissions due to their unique properties. The ability to incorporate functional moieties into peptides has created a new path for the development of smart nanomaterials with advanced functionalities. Peptide-based drug delivery systems, tissue engineering scaffolds, biosensors, and imaging agents are some of the promising applications of peptides in nanotechnology. However, several challenges remain, and further research is required to overcome these challenges and unlock the full potential of peptides in nanotechnology.

1.10 PRACTICE QUESTIONS

1. What are peptides and how do they differ from proteins in terms of size and structure?
2. How can peptides be synthesized and modified for use in nanotechnology applications?
3. What are some of the key properties of peptides that make them attractive for use in nanotechnology, such as biocompatibility and ease of functionalization?
4. What are some examples of nanotechnology applications that have utilized peptides, such as drug delivery or biosensors?
5. How do researchers ensure the stability and efficacy of peptide-based nanotechnology systems, and what challenges do they face in this area?

REFERENCES

1. Gentilucci, L.; De Marco, R.; Cerisoli, L., Chemical modifications designed to improve peptide stability: Incorporation of non-natural amino acids, pseudo-peptide bonds, and cyclization. *Current Pharmaceutical Design* 2010, 16 (28), 3185–3203.
2. Jakubke, H.-D.; Sewald, N., *Peptides from A to Z: A concise encyclopedia*. John Wiley & Sons: 2008.
3. Harish, V.; Tewari, D.; Gaur, M.; Yadav, A. B.; Swaroop, S.; Bechelany, M.; Barhoum, A., Review on nanoparticles and nanostructured materials: Bioimaging, biosensing, drug delivery, tissue engineering, antimicrobial, and agro-food applications. *Nanomaterials* **2022**, *12* (3), 457.
4. Sheppard, R., The fluorenylmethoxycarbonyl group in solid phase synthesis. *Journal of Peptide Science: An Official Publication of the European Peptide Society* 2003, 9 (9), 545–552.
5. Amblard, M.; Fehrentz, J.-A.; Martinez, J.; Subra, G., Methods and protocols of modern solid phase peptide synthesis. *Molecular Biotechnology* 2006, 33, 239–254.
6. Behrendt, R.; White, P.; Offer, J., Advances in Fmoc solid-phase peptide synthesis. *Journal of Peptide Science* 2016, 22 (1), 4–27.
7. Barhoum, A.; Pal, K.; Rahier, H.; Uludag, H.; Kim, I. S.; Bechelany, M., Nanofibers as new-generation materials: From spinning and nano-spinning fabrication techniques to emerging applications. *Applied Materials Today* **2019**, 17, 1–35.
8. Jeevanandam, J.; Barhoum, A.; Chan, Y. S.; Dufresne, A.; Danquah, M. K., Review on nanoparticles and nanostructured materials: History, sources, toxicity and regulations. *Beilstein Journal of Nanotechnology* 2018, 9 (1), 1050–1074.
9. Barhoum, A.; El-Maghrabi, H. H.; Nada, A. A.; Sayegh, S.; Roualdes, S.; Renard, A.; Iatsunskyi, I.; Coy, E.; Bechelany, M., Simultaneous hydrogen and oxygen evolution reactions using free-standing nitrogen-doped-carbon–Co/CoO x nanofiber electrodes decorated with palladium nanoparticles. *Journal of Materials Chemistry A* 2021, 9 (33), 17724–17739.
10. Kim, D.; Kim, J.; Park, Y. I.; Lee, N.; Hyeon, T., Recent development of inorganic nanoparticles for biomedical imaging. *ACS Central Science* 2018, 4 (3), 324–336.
11. Salatin, S.; Maleki Dizaj, S.; Yari Khosroushahi, A., Effect of the surface modification, size, and shape on cellular uptake of nanoparticles. *Cell Biology International* 2015, 39 (8), 881–890.
12. Tang, X.; Wippel, H. H.; Chavez, J. D.; Bruce, J. E., Crosslinking mass spectrometry: A link between structural biology and systems biology. *Protein Science* 2021, 30 (4), 773–784.

13. Habibi, N.; Kamaly, N.; Memic, A.; Shafiee, H., Self-assembled peptide-based nanostructures: Smart nanomaterials toward targeted drug delivery. *Nano Today* 2016, 11 (1), 41–60.
14. Ruoslahti, E., Peptides as targeting elements and tissue penetration devices for nanoparticles. *Advanced Materials* 2012, 24 (28), 3747–3756.
15. Saranya, S.; Yasuri, A.; Inoka, C. P.; Laksiri, W., Theranostic Nanomaterials to Overcome the Challenges in Peptide-basedCancer Therapy, *Current Bioactive Compounds* 2024, 20 (8), e220124225925. DOI: 10.2174/0115734072285630240110 115046
16. Wang, Y.; Li, S.; Wang, X.; Chen, Q.; He, Z.; Luo, C.; Sun, J., Smart transformable nanomedicines for cancer therapy. *Biomaterials* **2021**, *271*, 120737.
17. Chen, J.; Jiang, Z.; Zhang, Y. S.; Ding, J.; Chen, X., Smart transformable nanoparticles for enhanced tumor theranostics. *Applied Physics Reviews* 2021, 8 (4), 041321.
18. Thambi, T.; Deepagan, V.; Ko, H.; Lee, D. S.; Park, J. H., Bioreducible polymersomes for intracellular dual-drug delivery. *Journal of Materials Chemistry* 2012, 22 (41), 22028–22036.
19. Ghadiri, M. R.; Granja, J. R.; Milligan, R. A.; McRee, D. E.; Khazanovich, N., Self-assembling organic nanotubes based on a cyclic peptide architecture. *Nature* **1993**, *366* (6453), 324–327.
20. Smith, A., Does it have a sporting chance? *Chemistry International – Newsmagazine for IUPAC* **2006**, *28* (1), 8–9.
21. Visakhapatnam, P., Indian craftsmen, artisans used nanotech 2000 years ago. *Deccan Herald* 2008, 1.
22. Cai, W.; Shin, D.-W.; Chen, K.; Gheysens, O.; Cao, Q.; Wang, S. X.; Gambhir, S. S.; Chen, X., Peptide-labeled near-infrared quantum dots for imaging tumor vasculature in living subjects. *Nano Letters* 2006, 6 (4), 669–676.
23. Hulla, J.; Sahu, S.; Hayes, A., Nanotechnology: History and future. *Human & Experimental Toxicology* 2015, 34 (12), 1318–1321.
24. Feynman, R. P., There's plenty of room at the bottom: An invitation to enter a new field of physics. *Miniaturization, Reinhold* **1961,** 63–76.
25. Merrifield, R. B., Solid phase peptide synthesis. I. The synthesis of a tetrapeptide. *Journal of the American Chemical Society* 1963, 85 (14), 2149–2154.
26. Dong, J.; Liu, Y.; Cui, Y., Artificial metal–peptide assemblies: Bioinspired assembly of peptides and metals through space and across length scales. *Journal of the American Chemical Society* 2021, 143 (42), 17316–17336.
27. Zsigmondy, R., Colloids and the ultra microscope. *Journal of the American Chemical Society* 1909, 31 (8), 951–952.
28. Fanciullino, R.; Ciccolini, J., Liposome-encapsulated anticancer drugs: Still waiting for the magic bullet? *Current Medicinal Chemistry* 2009, 16 (33), 4361–4373.
29. Qi, G. B.; Gao, Y. J.; Wang, L.; Wang, H., Self-assembled peptide-based nanomaterials for biomedical imaging and therapy. *Advanced Materials* **2018**, *30* (22), 1703444.
30. Ochekpe, N. A.; Olorunfemi, P. O.; Ngwuluka, N. C., Nanotechnology and drug delivery part 1: Background and applications. *Tropical Journal of Pharmaceutical Research* **2009**, *8* (3).
31. Oh, J. K.; Drumright, R.; Siegwart, D. J.; Matyjaszewski, K., The development of microgels/nanogels for drug delivery applications. *Progress in Polymer Science* **2008**, *33* (4), 448–477.
32. Pearce, A. K.; Wilks, T. R.; Arno, M. C.; O'Reilly, R. K., Synthesis and applications of anisotropic nanoparticles with precisely defined dimensions. *Nature Reviews Chemistry* 2021, 5 (1), 21–45.
33. Sakala, G. P.; Reches, M., Peptide-based approaches to fight biofouling. *Advanced Materials Interfaces* **2018**, *5* (18), 1800073.

34. Gupta, A.; Bahal, R.; Gupta, M.; Glazer, P. M.; Saltzman, W. M., Nanotechnology for delivery of peptide nucleic acids (PNAs). *Journal of Controlled Release* 2016, 240, 302–311.
35. Panda, J. J.; Chauhan, V. S., Short peptide based self-assembled nanostructures: Implications in drug delivery and tissue engineering. *Polymer Chemistry* 2014, 5 (15), 4418–4436.
36. Rajagopal, K.; Schneider, J. P., Self-assembling peptides and proteins for nanotechnological applications. *Current Opinion in Structural Biology* 2004, 14 (4), 480–486.
37. Ariga, K., Nanoarchitectonics: What's coming next after nanotechnology? *Nanoscale Horizons* **2021**, *6* (5), 364–378.
38. Balzani, V., Nanoscience and nanotechnology: A personal view of a chemist. *Small* **2005**, *1* (3), 278–283.
39. Teo, B. K.; Sun, X., From top-down to bottom-up to hybrid nanotechnologies: Road to nanodevices. *Journal of Cluster Science* 2006, 17, 529–540.
40. Yadav, N.; Chauhan, M. K.; Chauhan, V. S., Short to ultrashort peptide-based hydrogels as a platform for biomedical applications. *Biomaterials Science* 2020, 8 (1), 84–100.
41. Desale, K.; Kuche, K.; Jain, S., Cell-penetrating peptides (CPPs): An overview of applications for improving the potential of nanotherapeutics. *Biomaterials Science* 2021, 9 (4), 1153–1188.
42. Bahar, A. A.; Ren, D., Antimicrobial peptides. *Pharmaceuticals* **2013**, *6* (12), 1543–1575.
43. Ray, A.; Nordén, B., Peptide nucleic acid (PNA): Its medical and biotechnical applications and promise for the future. *The FASEB Journal* 2000, 14 (9), 1041–1060.
44. Morgan, R. S.; Tatsch, C. E.; Gushard, R. H.; Mcadon, J. M.; Warme, P. K., Chains of alternating sulfur and Π-bonded atoms in eight small proteins. *International Journal of Peptide and Protein Research* 1978, 11 (3), 209–217.
45. Ulery, B. D.; Nair, L. S.; Laurencin, C. T., Biomedical applications of biodegradable polymers. *Journal of Polymer Science Part B: Polymer Physics* **2011**, *49* (12), 832–864.
46. Ariga, K.; Makita, T.; Ito, M.; Mori, T.; Watanabe, S.; Takeya, J., Review of advanced sensor devices employing nanoarchitectonics concepts. *Beilstein Journal of Nanotechnology* 2019, 10 (1), 2014–2030.
47. Ariga, K., Nanoarchitectonics: What's coming next after nanotechnology? *Nanoscale Horizons* **2021**, *6* (5), 364–378.
48. Kumar Malik, D.; Baboota, S.; Ahuja, A.; Hasan, S.; Ali, J., Recent advances in protein and peptide drug delivery systems. *Current Drug Delivery* 2007, 4 (2), 141–151.
49. Kostiainen, R.; Kotiaho, T.; Kuuranne, T.; Auriola, S., Liquid chromatography/atmospheric pressure ionization–mass spectrometry in drug metabolism studies. *Journal of Mass Spectrometry* 2003, 38 (4), 357–372.
50. Pavan, S.; Berti, F., Short peptides as biosensor transducers. *Analytical and Bioanalytical Chemistry* 2012, 402, 3055–3070.
51. Furth, M. E.; Atala, A.; Van Dyke, M. E., Smart biomaterials design for tissue engineering and regenerative medicine. *Biomaterials* **2007**, *28* (34), 5068–5073.
52. Malonis, R. J.; Lai, J. R.; Vergnolle, O., Peptide-based vaccines: Current progress and future challenges. *Chemical Reviews* 2019, 120 (6), 3210–3229.
53. Sánchez, A.; Vázquez, A., Bioactive peptides: A review. *Food Quality and Safety*, 2017, 1(1), 29–46.

2 Synthesis and characterization of peptides

2.1 PEPTIDE AND CHEMICAL SYNTHESIS

Peptide synthesis is the process of creating a peptide bond formed by the joining of two or more amino acids to form a peptide chain; this process is achieved through two main methods: chemical synthesis and biosynthesis.[1] In chemical synthesis, the amino acids are joined together using chemical reactions to form the peptide bond. Biosynthesis, on the other hand, involves the use of living cells to produce peptides.[2]

Characterization of peptides is an essential step in peptide synthesis. It involves the identification and quantification of the peptide, as well as the determination of its structure and biological activity. Various techniques are used in peptide characterization, including mass spectrometry, nuclear magnetic resonance (NMR) spectroscopy, high-performance liquid chromatography (HPLC), and circular dichroism (CD) spectroscopy.[3] Nevertheless, peptide synthesis and characterization are critical for understanding peptide biological action and developing therapeutic agents. These techniques enable researchers to create and study a wide range of peptides with various applications in medicine, biotechnology, and other fields.

2.2 BIOLOGICAL SYNTHESIS

The biological synthesis of proteins, also known as protein biosynthesis or translation, is a key mechanism that happens in all living cells both in eukaryotic cells and in prokaryotic cells. It is a significant process that occurs in all living cells using the information encoded in their DNA.[4] Protein synthesis involves two main steps: transcription and translation.

1. Transcription

    The protein synthesis is initiated by transcription, which is located in the cell nucleus in eukaryotic cells and the nucleoid region in prokaryotic cells.[5] During the transcription, the DNA molecule is unwound, and one of its strands serves as a template. RNA polymerase is the enzyme responsible for reading the DNA template strand and synthesizes a complementary RNA molecule, known as messenger RNA (mRNA). The mRNA molecule is synthesized in a 5'-to-3' direction and contains the genetic code for a specific protein.[6]

2. Translation

The transcription is continued by translation, which occurs in the cytoplasm in both prokaryotic and eukaryotic cells. During translation, the mRNA molecule leaves the nucleus and attaches to ribosomes in the cytoplasm. While the ribosomes read the mRNA sequence in groups of three nucleotides called codons. Each codon codes for a specific amino acid. Transfer RNA (tRNA) molecules carry the corresponding amino acids to the ribosome.[7]

The tRNA molecules have an anticodon region that can base-pair with the mRNA codon, ensuring the correct amino acid is added to the growing protein chain (Table 2.1).[8] The ribosome catalyzes the creation of peptide bonds between neighboring amino acids as it advances along the mRNA, resulting in the production of a polypeptide chain. This procedure is repeated until an mRNA stop codon is reached, signifying the end of protein synthesis. The newly synthesized polypeptide chain then folds into its functional three-dimensional structure, which is critical for its biological activity.[9]

The sequence of codons in the mRNA influences the sequence of amino acids in the polypeptide chain, which is primarily identified through the DNA sequence of the gene. The metabolism of protein synthesis is highly regulated and plays a

TABLE 2.1
The amino acids specified by each mRNA codon. Multiple codons can code for the same amino acid

UUU-Phe	UCU-Ser	UAU-Tyr	UGU-Cys
UUC-Phe	UCC-Ser	UAC-Tyr	UGC-Cys
UUA-Leu	UCA-Ser	UAA-Stop	UGA-Stop
UUG-Leu	UCG-Ser	UAG-Stop	UGG-Trp
CUU-Leu	CCU-Pro	CAU-His	CGU-Arg
CUC-Leu	CCC-Pro	CAC-His	CGC-Arg
CUA-Leu	CCA-Pro	CAA-Gla	CGA-Arg
CUG-Lleu	CCG-Pro	CAG-Gla	CGG-Arg
AUU-Ile	AUC-Thr	AAU-Asn	AGU-Ser
AUC-Ile	ACC-Thr	AAC-Asn	AGC-Ser
AUA-Ile	ACA-Thr	AAA-Lys	AGA-Arg
AUG-Met start	ACG-Thr	AAG-Lys	AGG-Arg
GUU-Val	GCU-Ala	GAU-Asp	GGU-Gly
GUC-Val	GCC-Ala	GAC-Asp	GGC-Gly
GUA-Val	GCA-Ala	GAA-Glu	GGA-Gly
GUG-Val	GCG-Ala	GAG-Glu	GGG-Gly

vital role in the functioning of cells, as proteins are essential for various cellular functions, including enzymatic reactions, structural support, and cell signaling. Any errors or mutations in the protein synthesis process can lead to genetic diseases or cellular dysfunction.[10]

Ribosomal and non-ribosomal synthesis are two processes engaged in the synthesis of peptides and proteins. There are differences in their mechanisms, locations, and the types of molecules involved.[11] Here's an overview of both ribosomal and non-ribosomal peptide/protein synthesis.

2.3 RIBOSOMAL SYNTHESIS

Ribosomal synthesis occurs on ribosomes. In eukaryotic cells the ribosmomes are found in the cytoplasm, while in prokaryotic cells they are located in the cytoplasm or attached to the cell membrane. However, ribosomes are complex structures made up of ribosomal RNA (rRNA) and proteins, which serve as the machinery for protein synthesis.[12] While mRNA molecules are formed by ribosomes that read the genetic information encoded in mRNA (Figure 2.1) to synthesize proteins, tRNA molecules transport amino acids from the cell to the ribosome, matching them with the codons on the mRNA. Ribosomal synthesis is part of the process of translation, where the ribosome reads the mRNA and assembles amino acids in the correct sequence to form a polypeptide chain. The ribosome moves along the mRNA, and each codon on the mRNA is recognized by a complementary anticodon on the tRNA, ensuring the proper amino acid is added to the growing polypeptide chain. The ribosome continues this process until it reaches a stop codon, at which point protein synthesis is terminated.[13]

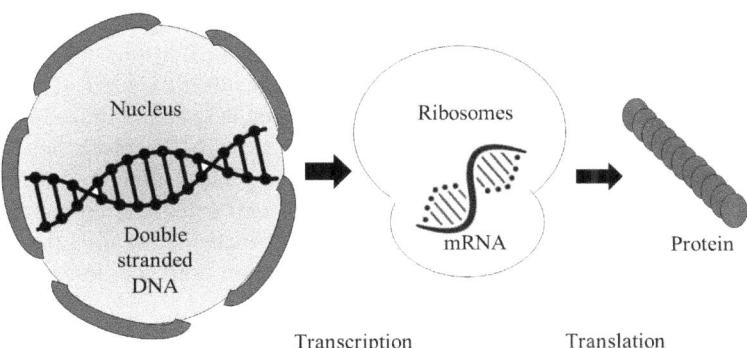

FIGURE 2.1 Schematic diagram of mRNA moving into the cytoplasm from the nucleus after the transcription process inside the nucleus membrane and assembling into a specific sequence of amino acids to form the protein via a process called translation. The process that uses ribosomal is called ribosomal synthesis.

2.4 NON-RIBOSOMAL SYNTHESIS

Non-ribosomal synthesis occurs in specialized cellular structures known as non-ribosomal peptide synthetases (NRPSs) or non-ribosomal peptide assembly lines. NRPSs are large multi-enzyme complexes responsible for non-ribosomal peptide synthesis. They are found in bacteria and fungi.[14] Instead of relying on mRNA and ribosomes, NRPSs directly incorporate amino acids into the growing peptide chain. NRPS complexes often include various domains that perform functions like amino acid activation, condensation, and modification. Non-ribosomal synthesis involves a modular and template-driven process, where each module of the NRPS complex is responsible for incorporating a specific amino acid into the peptide chain.[15]

The process is not guided by mRNA and ribosomes but is determined by the specific organization and domains within the NRPS complex. Non-ribosomal synthesis is common for the production of non-ribosomal peptides, which often have roles in secondary metabolite production, antibiotics, and other specialized functions.[16] Non-ribosomal synthesis is particularly important in order to generate secondary metabolites in microorganisms, such as antibiotics (e.g., penicillin) and toxins (e.g., cyanotoxins). These compounds are typically synthesized using NRPSs.[17]

Thus, ribosomal synthesis is the more common and widely known process for protein synthesis, occurring on ribosomes in all living cells. Non-ribosomal synthesis, on the other hand, is a specialized mechanism primarily found in microorganisms for the production of non-ribosomal peptides with various biological functions.

2.5 CHEMICAL SYNTHESIS OF PEPTIDES

Chemical synthesis is a widely used method for producing high-purity and quantity peptides. In this chapter, we will discuss the chemical synthesis of peptides, including the different methods and techniques involved. Chemical synthesis of peptides involves the formation of peptide bonds between amino acids using chemical reactions.[18] The process typically starts with the protection of the N-terminal and C-terminal of the amino acids to prevent unwanted side reactions.[19] The protected amino acids are then activated using a coupling reagent, such as N,N'-diisopropylcarbodiimide (DIC), and reacted containing the following amino acid in the chain. This process is repeated until the desired peptide chain is formed.[20]

There are two main methods of chemical peptide synthesis: solution-phase synthesis and solid-phase synthesis.[21] The protected amino acids are dissolved in a solvent during solution-phase synthesis, and the reactions take place in the solution. This method is suitable for producing small peptides but becomes increasingly challenging for larger peptides due to difficulties in purification and separation.[22]

Solid-phase synthesis, on the other hand, uses a solid substrate, commonly resin, to which the first amino acid is linked.[21] The reactions are then carried out on the solid support, allowing for easy purification and separation. This method is particularly suitable for producing larger peptides and is commonly employed in industrial-scale manufacturing of peptides.

One of the challenges in chemical peptide synthesis is the development of peptide bonds between amino acids. This reaction is slow and typically requires the use of coupling reagents to increase the reaction rate.[23] However, these reagents might potentially result in unfavorable side effects, such as racemization and epimerization, which might decrease ultimate product yield and purity.

To address these issues, scholars have devised a variety of solutions and techniques for improving the efficiency and purity of peptide synthesis. For example, the use of pre-activated amino acids, such as N-hydroxysuccinimide (NHS) esters, can improve the reaction rate and reduce side reactions.[24] Other techniques, such as microwave-assisted peptide synthesis[23] and flow chemistry,[25] have also been developed to improve the speed and efficiency of peptide synthesis.

In addition to the synthesis of peptides, characterization is also an essential step in peptide research. Various techniques are used to characterize peptides, including mass spectrometry, NMR spectroscopy, and HPLC. These procedures enable researchers to determine the peptide's purity, structure, and biological activity.[26]

2.5.1 SOLID-PHASE PEPTIDE SYNTHESIS

Solid-phase peptide synthesis (SPPS) is a widely used method for the chemical synthesis of peptides, which are short chains comprising amino acids bonded together by peptide bonds. It allows for the rapid and efficient synthesis of peptides with high purity and precision, making it a dominant tool in peptide research, drug discovery, and biotechnology.

In SPPS, the peptide chain is constructed stepwise on a solid support, typically a resin, with each amino acid added in a protected form. Coupling reactions are used to link the amino acids together, and deprotection steps are used to eliminate the protecting groups, allowing the peptide to elongate. The final peptide product can be cleaved from the resin and purified for further analysis and application. SPPS has undergone significant advancements since Merrifield's inception in the 1960s,[27] including the development of new resins and protecting groups, as well as the use of automation and computer-assisted design to streamline and optimize the synthesis process. In this chapter, we share the theoretical basis, step-by-step protocol, modifications and variations, limitations, and future directions of SPPS, providing a comprehensive overview of this important peptide synthesis method.

Peptide bonds link amino acids together by forming one amino acid's carboxyl group (COOH) and another amino acid's amino group (NH_2), resulting in the production of another amino acid, causing the formation of a carbon-nitrogen bond and the release of a water molecule.[28] The reaction is catalyzed by enzymes

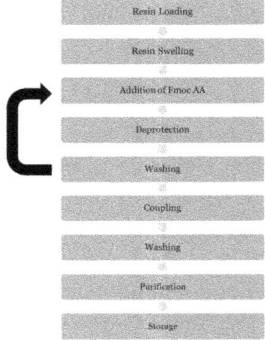

FIGURE 2.2 Overall stages of the SPSS.

called ribosomes in the case of protein synthesis,[29] but chemical methods are needed for the synthesis of peptides in the laboratory.

The theoretical basis of SPPS lies in the principles of peptide bond formation and protecting group strategy, which is essential for sequential peptide chain construction on a solid support. SPPS has undergone significant advancements since its introduction in the 1960s, including the development of new resins, protecting groups, coupling reagents, and deprotection methods, which have improved the efficiency, selectivity, and purity of the synthesis process.

SPPS is a powerful technique used for the efficient synthesis of peptides. Here is a step-by-step protocol for SPPS (Figure 2.2):

2.5.1.1 Solid support and linkers

In SPPS, the peptide chain is gathered stepwise on a solid support, typically a resin, with each amino acid added in a protected form. The resin is connected to its initial amino acid through a linker, which allows for the attachment of subsequent amino acids.[27,30] The linker is typically composed of a hydrophilic spacer and a reactive group that can be used for coupling with the amino acid.[31] The linker can also be modified to control the peptide dissociation from resin at the final stage of synthesis. This specifically manufactured insoluble polymer resin that, under some circumstances, links to the initial amino acid C-terminus and, under additional circumstances, allows the last peptide chain to be separated from the structure of the resin after synthesis.[32] Choose the appropriate resin for the synthesis, based on the desired C-terminal modification and compatibility with the amino acid building blocks. Commonly used resins include polystyrene (PS), Wang resin, and Rink amide resin (Table 2.2).[33]

Figures 2.3–2.7 are schematic diagrams of different types of resins and links.

Here are a few more examples of the resins and linkers that can be used according to our requirements such as grafted polyethylene glycol (PEG) resin, TentaGel resin, and PS resin, cross-linked with divinylbenzene (DVB), which are considerably inexpensive standard resins for routine syntheses.[38,39] ChemMatrix resin,

Synthesis and characterization of peptides

TABLE 2.2
The different types of resins and links used

Types	Specification	Two-dimensional structure	Reference
Rink Amide (Methylbenzhydrylamine) MBHA resin	Rink Amide MBHA resins are designed for the Fmoc method of C-terminal amide synthesis. Norleucine and aminomethyl PS are connected in these resins. The Fmoc-Rinkamid (4-(2′,4′-dimethoxyphenyl-Fmoc-amino methyl)-phenoxy)-functional group is very sensitive to the effects of acids and is bonded to PS using 1% DVB. Because of this, , the last peptide is exceedingly rapidly extracted from these resins substantially diluted by acid, such as 1% TFA/DCM or 10% AcOH (acetic acid)/DCM, making it to be user-friendly and commonly used material.	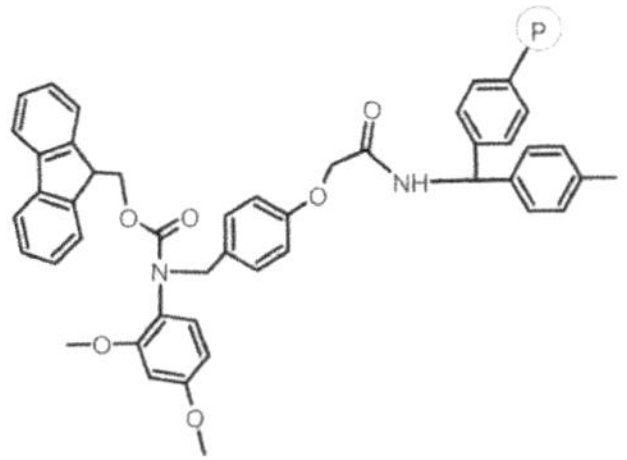 FIGURE 2.3 Chemical Structure of Rink Amide MBHA resin	32
Wang resin	Obtaining the C-terminal functional group as carboxy, the linker in Wang resins is 4-(hydroxymethyl)phenoxyacetic acid residue that is PEG-adhered to PS, silica gel, or other supports that permit the synthesis of lengthy peptides. This linker is resilient under basic circumstances but easily cleaves under acidic conditions with 90% TFA to yield a peptide acid. The initial amino acid is generally coupled to the linker using 4-(dimethylamino)pyridine (Dmap) as a catalyst. This process can have unwanted adverse reactions and be dangerous.	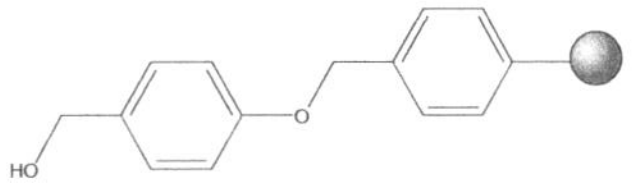 FIGURE 2.4 Chemical Structure of Wang resin	32

2-Chlorotrityl linker

The C-terminal function is protected by carboxyl. It arrives connected to the initial amino acid and is very acid labile. It can be broken down with a low-TFA solution and is advised for the production of peptides with C-terminal Pro or Cys.

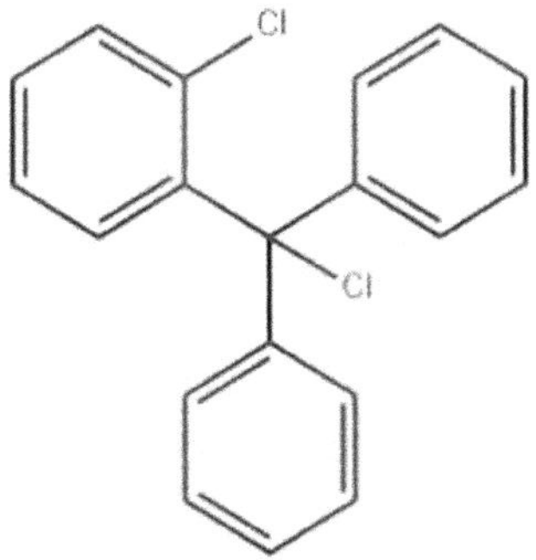

FIGURE 2.5 Chemical Structure of 2-Chlorotrityl linker

HMBA linker

The linker has global applicability. The category of C-terminal functionality is determined by the cleavage reaction, such as amide, carboxyl, modified amide, hydrazide, ester, and alcohol.

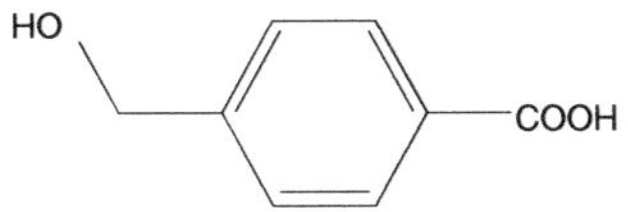

FIGURE 2.6 Chemical Structure of HMBA linker

Sieber amide linker

While the C-terminal functions as an amide, it is very acid labile and yields protected peptide fragments after cleavage in a low-TFA solution.

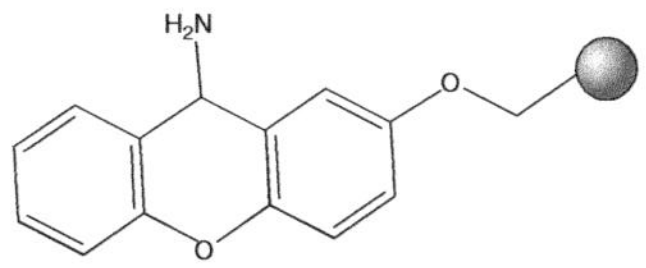

FIGURE 2.7 Chemical Structure of Sieber amide linker

NovaPEG resin, and CLEAR resin are resins with strong swelling capability in SPPS solvents, which are very valuable for demanding sequence applications.[40]

2.5.1.2 Protecting groups

Protecting the N-terminus of the resin with a suitable protecting group is vital, such as the Boc (*tert*-butoxycarbonyl) or Fmoc (9-fluorenylmethyloxycarbonyl) group.[41] The protective group is chosen based on the resin and amino acids utilized in the synthesis. One of the challenges in peptide synthesis is the tendency of the reaction to proceed in the reverse direction, leading to the cleavage of the peptide bond and the reformation of the amino acid starting materials. This can occur due to the electrophilicity of the carbonyl carbon in the peptide bond which can attract nucleophiles such as water and hydronium ions.[42] To prevent this, the amino and carboxyl groups of the amino acids are protected with specific chemical groups during the synthesis process.[43]

Protecting groups are temporary modifications to the amino acid functional groups that can be added and removed as needed during peptide synthesis. Protective units are employed to prevent undesirable interactions between functional groups (Figure 2.8), while still allowing selective reactions to occur at specific sites. For example, the amino group of an amino acid can be protected with a group such as the Boc group, which is removed by acid treatment. The carboxyl group can be protected with a group such as the benzyl (Bzl) group, which is removed by hydrogenation.

Tables 2.3 and 2.4 reveal protecting groups and their significance.

Additional α-amino protecting groups include benzyloxycarbonyl (Z)[64,65] and allyloxycarbonyl (Alloc) (Tables 2.5 and 2.6)[65,66]

2.5.2 COUPLING REACTION

Coupling reagents are utilized to combat the high activation energy for the creation of amide bonds between amino acid amine and carboxylate groups. To

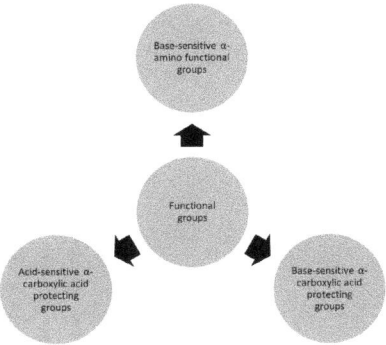

FIGURE 2.8 The conditions for protection and removal are presented to assist the reader in finding appropriate reagents based on their unique needs.

TABLE 2.3
α-Amino-protecting groups removed by base (base-sensitive α-amino functional groups)

Name and structure	Protection conditions	Removal conditions	Reference
Fmoc	1. Fmoc-Cl, in H$_2$O-dioxane (3:1), Na$_2$CO$_3$ 2. Fmoc-Osu, in dioxane-H$_2$O (1:1)/ NaHCO$_3$ 3. (N-[(9H-fluoren-9-yl)methoxy] carbonyloxy) picolinimidoyl cyanide (Fmoc-Oxyma), in acetone-H$_2$O (1:1), NaHCO$_3$	Solid phase: 1. 20% 4-MePip in DMF 2. 1–5% DBU in DMF 3. 50% Morpholine in DMF (1:1) 4. 50% Ethanolamine in DCM 5. 2% HOBt, 2% hexamethyleneimine, 25% N-methylpyrrolidine in DMSO-NMP (1:1) Solution phase: 1. NH$_3$ (10 h) 2. Morpholine or piperdine in organic solvents 3. 10% DEA, DMA (2 h) 4. Polymeric secondary amines (i.e., piperidine, piperazines) in organic solvents	45,46
(1,1-Dioxobenzo[*b*]thiophene-2-yl) methyloxycarbonyl (Bsmoc)	NHS, (CH$_3$)3SiCl, NMM, DCM, reflux	1. 2–5% Piperidine in DMF 2. 2% Tris(2-aminoethyl)amine (TAEA) in DCM	47,48
1,1-Dioxonaphtho[1,2-*b*]thiophene2-yl) methyloxycarbonyl (α-Nsmoc)	(CH$_3$)3SiCl, Diisopropylethylamine (DIEPA), DCM, reflux	1. 2–5% Piperidine in DMF	49
1-(4,4-Dimethyl-2-6-dioxocyclohex1-ylidene)ethyl (Dde)	2-(1-Hydroxy-3-methylbutylidene)-5,5-dimethyl cyclohexane-1,3-dione, DIEPA, MeOH, reflux	1. 2% N$_2$H$_4$ in DMF	50
Tetrachloro-phthaloyl (TCP)	4,5,6,7-Tetrachloroisobenzofuran-1, 3-dione, AcOH, reflux	1. Hydrazine/DMF (3:17), 40°C, 1 h 2. 0.5% Ethylenediamine in DMF, 50·°C, 30 min	51,52
2-(4-Sulfophenylsulfonyl) ethoxycarbonyl (Sps)	4-Nitrophenylchloroformate, conc: H$_2$SO$_4$/Ac$_2$O, H$_2$O$_2$/TFA	1. 5% Aqueous Na$_2$CO$_3$	53
Trifluoroacetyl (tfa)	1. Ethyl 2,2,2- 2. trifluoroacetate, Et$_3$N, MeOH, rt. 2. TFAA, DCM, 0 °C to rt.	1. NaOH (0.2 N), 10 min 2. 1 M Aqueous piperidine 3. NaBH$_4$ in ethanol 4. K$_2$CO$_3$, H$_2$O, MeOH	54,55

TABLE 2.4
Sensitive α-amino functional groups

Name and structure	Protection conditions	Removal conditions	Reference
Trityl (Trt)	Trityl chloride, Et₃N, DCM	1. 1% TFA in DCM 2. HOBt (0.1 M) in TFE 3. 0.2% TFA, 1% H₂O in DCM 4. 3% TCA in DCM 5. 10 eq Li, 0.2 eq 6. Naphthalene, THF	51,56
2-(4-Biphenyl) isopropoxycarbonyl (Bpoc)	Carbonic acid, 1-[1,10-biphenyl]-4-yl-1-methylethyl phenyl ester, CHCl₃, 50 C	1. 0.5% TFA in DCM	57,58
2-Nitrophenylsulfenyl (Nps)	NaOH (2 N) or NaHCO₃, 1,4-dioxane, or H₂O	1. Dilute solutions of CH₃CO₂H/ HCl/CHCl₃ 2. Raney Ni in DMF CH₃CO₂H in MeOH, 2-mercaptopyridine in DMF or DCM	59,60
tert-Butyloxycarbonyl (Boc)	1. Boc2O, Et₃N, THF, H₂O 2. Boc2O, MAP, CAN 3. Boc2O, HFIP	1. HCl (4 M) in dioxane 2. 25–50% TFA in DCM 3. Methanesulfonic acid (2M) in dioxane 4. Trimethylsilyl chloride (1M), phenol in DCM	61–63

TABLE 2.5
Base sensitive

Name and structure	Protection conditions	Removal conditions	Reference
9-Fluorenylmethyl (Fm)	9-Fluorenylmethanol, DCC, DMAP	1. 10% N-methylcyclohexylamine in DCM 2. 20% 4-MePip in DMF	48,46
Methyl or ethyl	Methanol or ethanol, H_2SO_4 (cat.) or Para-Toluenesulfonic Acid (PTSA)	1. Aqueous NaOH or KOH 2. $AlCl_3$/N,N-dimethylaniline (DMA), DCM	67,68
Carbamoylmethyl (cam)	2-Chloroacetamide, Cs_2CO_3, EtOH, H_2O, DMF	1. NaOH (0.5 N) or Na_2CO_3 (0.5 N) in a mixture of DMF/H_2O (3:1)	67,69

TABLE 2.6
Acid-sensitive α-carboxylic acid protecting groups

Name and structure	Protection conditions	Removal conditions	Reference
2-Phenylisopropyl (2-Phi Pr)	2-Phenylpropan-2-ol, NaH, CCl_3CN, THF, 0 °C	1. 4% TFA in DCM	70
2-Chlorotrityl (2-Cl-Trt)	DIEPA, 2-Cl-Trt, DCM	1. 1% TFA in DCM	71
tert-Butyl (^{t}Bu)	^{t}BuOH, Et_3N, DCC, DMAP, DCM	1. 50–90% TFA in DCM 2. HCl (4 N) in 1,4-dioxane 3. ZnBr, DCM	72

couple the first amino acid to the resin using a coupling reagent, such as HATU (O-(7-azabenzotriazol-1-yl)-N,N,N',N'-tetramethyluronium hexafluorophosphate), HBTU (2-(1H-benzotriazol-1-yl)-1,1,3,3-tetramethylaminium hexafluorophosphate), or DIC is used and its vital to form a peptide bond, the carboxylic acid moiety of one amino acid should be activated with specific reagents as above. The amino acid is activated with a base, such as N,N-diisopropylethylamine (DIPEA) or N-methylmorpholine (NMM), and mixed with the coupling reagent N,N-dimethylformamide (DMF) or dichloromethane (DCM), which are appropriate solvents. The coupling reaction is carried out for several hours at room temperature or a slightly elevated temperature, depending on the coupling efficiency.

The coupling reaction in SPPS is completed using a carbodiimide coupling reagent, such as dicyclohexylcarbodiimide (DCC), which activates the carboxyl group of the amino acid and facilitates the nucleophilic attack of the amino group of the incoming amino acid. The coupling reaction is performed in the presence

Synthesis and characterization of peptides 27

of a base, such as N,N-diisopropylethylamine (DIPEA), which neutralizes the acid by-product and promotes the formation of the peptide bond. After the coupling reaction, any unreacted carboxyl groups are capped with a blocking reagent, such as acetic anhydride, to prevent unwanted reactions.

One of the challenges in SPPS is the need to overcome steric hindrance during peptide elongation. The protected amino acids get larger as the peptide chain increases and can obstruct the coupling interaction by binding to the entering amino acid. This can result in incomplete coupling and racemization. This may jeopardize the final peptide product's quality and yield. Several solutions have been explored to enhance the coupling efficiency and minimize racemization, including the use of pre-activated amino acid derivatives, coupling additives, and racemization-suppressing reagents.[44]

Pre-activated amino acid derivatives, such as the N-(1-(4,4-dimethyl-2, 6-dioxocyclohex-1-ylidene)ethyl)-N-methylamino)pyridinium tetrafluoroborate (DMAP-BF$_4$), might increase reaction pace and productivity of the coupling reaction by activating the carboxyl group and making it more nucleophilic.[73] Coupling additives, such as 1-hydroxybenzotriazole (HOBt), can also enhance via maintaining the coupling reaction's efficiency and selectivity activated carboxylate intermediate and suppressing racemization.[74] Racemization may take place at the C-terminal amino acid residue during a coupling process caused by -hydrogen ionization and the creation of an oxazolone intermediate. Racemization-suppressing reagents, such as 2-(6-chloro-1H-benzotriazole-1-yl)-1,1,3,3-tetramethylaminium hexafluorophosphate (HCTU), can prevent the racemization of chiral amino acids during the coupling reaction, resulting in increased quality and yield of the end peptide product.[75]

2.5.3 Deprotection

The process is repeated until the full-length peptide sequence is obtained, at which point the product is cleaved from the solid resin, and the side chain protecting groups are deprotected. Deprotection is another important step in SPPS, which involves the elimination of the amino and carboxyl protective groups to expose the reactive functional groups for the next coupling reaction. The deprotection step is typically carried out using specific reagents and conditions that are compatible with the resin and the protecting groups used in the synthesis. For example, the Boc protecting group may be eliminated using trifluoroacetic acid (TFA) in the presence of scavengers such as triisopropylsilane (TIS) to prevent side reactions, while the Bzl protecting group can be terminated through hydrogenation with palladium on carbon (Pd/C) in the presence of a hydrogen gas source. If Fmoc protection was used for the N-terminus, the Fmoc group is removed using a base, such as piperidine or N-methylmorpholine, in a suitable solvent, such as DMF or DCM. The deprotection step is typically carried out for several minutes, depending on the efficiency of the deprotection.[71]

Let's check the following steps to complete the cycle:

Amino acid coupling: Couple the next amino acid to the resin using a similar procedure as step 3. Repeat steps 4 and 5 until the desired peptide sequence is synthesized.

C-terminal deprotection: After the last amino acid is coupled, remove the C-terminal protecting group using a suitable reagent, such as TFA or HF (hydrogen fluoride), when scavengers such as thioanisole or ethanedithiol are present.[76] The deprotection step is typically carried out for several hours, depending on the resin and the protecting group used.

Peptide cleavage and purification: The last procedure in SPPS is to separate the peptide from the resin and purify the peptide product. The peptide can be sliced from the resin using specific cleavage reagents and conditions, such as TFA, which can also remove any remaining protecting groups. After cleavage, the peptide product could be purified with various chromatography techniques, such as reversed-phase HPLC (RP-HPLC), which separates the peptide based on its hydrophobicity and charge.[26]

The use of modern coupling reagents, protecting groups, and deprotection methods has significantly improved the efficiency and speed of SPPS. Additionally, advancements in automation and robotics have made SPPS an increasingly attractive option for large-scale peptide production.

However, SPPS is not without its challenges. One major issue is the production of by-products, which can reduce the end yield and purity. For example, incomplete coupling can lead to truncated peptides, while incomplete deprotection can result in a mixture of partially protected peptides.[77] Side reactions such as racemization could take place in the amino acid coupling stage, leading to the formation of diastereomers.[78,79] These challenges can be mitigated through careful selection of reagents, optimization of reaction conditions, and monitoring of reaction progress.

Another important consideration in SPPS is the choosing of suitable resins and protective groups. The choice of resin will depend on the desired C-terminal modification, as well as the compatibility with the amino acid stacks. For example, Wang resin is commonly used for the synthesis of peptides with a free C-terminus, while Rink amide resin is ideal for the production of peptides with an amide C-terminus. The choice of protecting group will depend on the amino acid utilized and the intended peptide sequence.[31]

Despite its challenges, SPPS has become a widely used technique in the realm of peptide synthesis, enabling the rapid manufacturing of peptides for several purposes, including drug development and discovery, biotechnology, and chemical biology. As the field continues to advance, new developments in SPPS will likely further improve its efficiency, speed, and versatility.

2.5.4 NEW TRENDS IN SPPS

The versatility of SPPS is enhanced through the use of modifications and variations that allow for the inclusion of various functional groups, modifications, and labeling tags. In this part, we will discover some of the modifications and variations of SPPS that have been developed over the years.

One common modification of SPPS is the use of orthogonal protecting groups. This entails using different protective groups for the same functional group, allowing for the sequential introduction of different functional groups into the peptide. This is particularly beneficial for the synthesis of peptides with multiple modifications, as it enables the selective introduction of each modification without affecting the others. A thiol group, for example, can be introduced to selectively achieve using an orthogonal protecting group approach, allowing for the incorporation of disulfide bonds in the peptide.[80]

Another variation of SPPS is the use of ligation strategies. This involves the synthesis of two or more peptide fragments separately, followed by their ligation to form a larger peptide. This approach can be useful for creating significantly big peptides or proteins that are difficult to synthesize by SPPS alone.[81] Chemical ligation, expressed protein ligation, and native chemical ligation (NCL) are all techniques for achieving ligation.

A peptide fragment containing a C-terminal thioester and a second fragment with an N-terminal cysteine are used in chemical ligation. The two fragments can be selectively ligated in the presence of a thiol catalyst, creating a bond between the two sequences of fragments. Expressed protein ligation, on the other hand, involves the use of recombinant protein fragments that are expressed *in vivo*, followed by their purification and ligation *in vitro*. A peptide fragment with an N-terminal cysteine and a second fragment with a C-terminal thioester is used in NCL, which can be selectively ligated using a thiol catalyst.

In addition to ligation strategies, SPPS can also be modified to include unnatural amino acids. This can be accomplished by using chemically modified amino acids or nonnatural amino acid analogs. Chemically modified by altering the side chain of a natural amino acid, modified amino acids can be created, while nonnatural amino acid analogs can be synthesized by modifying the peptide backbone itself.[82] The incorporation of nonnatural amino acids can enhance the biological activity or stability of the peptide or allow for the introduction of new chemical properties.

Finally, SPPS can be modified to incorporate posttranslational modifications (PTMs). PTMs are chemical modifications that occur after translation and can include phosphorylation, glycosylation, and acetylation, among others. The incorporation of PTMs into peptides can be challenging, as the modifications can be sensitive to the conditions used in SPPS. However, modifications such as phosphorylation and glycosylation can be achieved through the use of pre-activated sugars or phosphorylated amino acid derivatives.[83]

Thus, the modifications and variations of SPPS have greatly expanded its versatility and allowed for the synthesis of peptides with a diverse functional group, modifications, and labeling tags. Orthogonal protecting groups, ligation strategies, integration of nonnatural amino acids, and incorporation of PTMs are just a few of the modifications that have been developed to enhance the capabilities of SPPS. These modifications have opened up new avenues to create peptides with improved biological effectiveness, rigidity, and chemical characteristics. As the field continues to advance, new modifications and variations of SPPS will likely be developed, further expanding its utility in the synthesis of complex peptides and proteins.

2.5.5 LIMITATIONS OF SPPS

SPPS has revolutionized the field of peptide synthesis, enabling the efficient and quick synthesis of high-purity and yield peptides. It has a diverse range of applications in a variety of industries, including biochemistry, pharmacology, and materials science, while its limitations have been marked as well.

1. Length: SPPS is limited in its ability to synthesize long peptides or proteins. The yield of the synthesis diminishes as the length of the peptide rises, and the risk of side reactions and aggregation increases.[84]
2. Complexity: SPPS might be challenging to work with when attempting to synthesize peptides containing PTMs or nonstandard amino acids. The SPPS criteria may be incompatible with the stability of the modification or the nonstandard amino acid.[85]
3. Cost: SPPS requires expensive equipment and reagents, which can be a limiting factor for some researchers or institutions.[86]
4. Scale-up: SPPS is typically performed on a small scale, making it difficult to synthesize large quantities of peptides. Scale-up can be challenging, and the yield and purity of the peptide may be compromised.[86]
5. Purification: After the synthesis, the peptide must be purified to remove any impurities or side products. Purification can be challenging, particularly for complex peptides, and may require multiple rounds of chromatography.[87]

SPPS has numerous applications in various fields, including drug discovery, immunology, materials science, and structural biology. However, it also has its limitations, including the length and complexity of the peptides that can be synthesized. While the expenses of the instruments and reagents, the difficulties of purification, and scale-up excute challenges in using SPSS. As the field continues to advance, new modifications and variations of SPPS may be developed to overcome some of these limitations, further expanding its applications in peptide synthesis and related fields.

Future research in the field of SPPS is focused on addressing these limitations and developing new strategies for peptide synthesis. One promising direction is the creation of new strong supports and linkers that can improve the efficiency and yield of SPPS, as well as the production of longer and more complex peptides. In addition, the incorporation of novel amino acid analogs and nonnatural SPPS can be expanded by converting amino acids into peptides and enabling the production of peptides with unique properties and functions.

Overall, the continued advancement of SPPS techniques and technologies will play a critical role in the creation of new therapeutic agents, biomaterials, and

Synthesis and characterization of peptides

bioanalytical tools, as well as expanding our consideration of the structure and function of peptides in biological systems.

2.5.6 Liquid/Solution-Phase Peptide Synthesis

Liquid/solution-phase peptide synthesis (LPPS) is a method for synthesizing peptides in solution rather than on a solid support.[88] In LPPS, the peptide is formed by adding one amino acid at a time to a developing chain of amino acids in solution. This is in contrast to SPPS, where the peptide is synthesized on a solid support, such as a resin.

In LPPS, the amino acids are activated by a coupling reagent and then supplied to the developing peptide chain. The side-chain protecting groups are typically acid-labile in LPPS, which allows for their removal under mildly acidic conditions without affecting the peptide backbone.[89]

LPPS can be advantageous over SPPS for certain peptide sequences or when working with difficult amino acids or modified peptides. It can also be used to synthesize stronger peptides or even proteins, which can be more challenging with SPPS.[90] However, it can be more time-consuming and can require more synthetic steps than SPPS. Additionally, LPPS can suffer from poor yields due to the complexity in terms of the reaction parameters and the difficulty of purifying peptides from solution.[91]

LPPS is a method to synthesize peptides in solution rather than on a solid support. In LPPS, the peptide is built up by adding one amino acid at a time to a growing chain in solution. A coupling reagent is used to activate the amino acids before they are introduced to the developing peptide chain.[92] In acids, side-chain protecting groups are acid-labile in LPPS, which allows for their removal under mildly acidic conditions without affecting the peptide backbone.[93]

The development of LPPS is traced all the way back to the 1960s when the first reports on solution-phase peptide synthesis were published. Early attempts at LPPS were often plagued by low yields and difficulties in purification, and as a result, SPPS quickly became the dominant method for peptide synthesis.

However, in the 1980s, advancements in the development of coupling reagents and amino acid derivatives led to renewed interest in LPPS.[94] Today, LPPS is a recognized peptide synthesis process that is frequently employed in the pharmaceutical field and academic research.

2.5.6.1 Advantages and disadvantages of LPPS compared to SPPS

One advantage of LPPS over SPPS is that it enables the production of longer-sized peptides or even proteins, which can be more challenging with SPPS. Additionally, LPPS can be advantageous for certain peptide sequences or when working with difficult amino acids or modified peptides.

However, LPPS can be more time-consuming and can require more synthetic steps than SPPS. Additionally, LPPS can suffer from poor yields due to the complexity given the reaction conditions and the difficulty of separating peptides from the solution. Overall, the choice between LPPS and SPPS depends on the specific peptide sequence being synthesized and the desired outcome of the synthesis. LPPS is a versatile method of synthesizing peptides in solution.

2.5.6.2 Step-by-step protocol of LPPS

The chemistry of LPPS involves several key steps, including activation of amino acids, coupling reactions, use of protecting groups, and side-chain deprotection.

A. Activation of amino acids

In LPPS, before amino acids can be linked to the developing peptide chain, they must be activated. This is typically done by reacting the amino acid with a coupling reagent, such as DCC or DIC, to form an active ester intermediate. The activated amino acid is next linked to the expanding peptide chain.[95]

B. Coupling reagents

Coupling reagents are essential in LPPS for the activation of amino acids and the formation of peptide bonds. In addition to DCC and DIC, other commonly used coupling reagents in LPPS include HBTU (O-(benzotriazol-1-yl)-N,N,N',N'-tetramethyluronium hexafluorophosphate), HATU, and TBTU (O-(benzotriazol-1-yl)-N,N,N',N'-tetramethyl uronium tetrafluoroborate).[95]

C. Protecting groups

In LPPS, protecting groups are used to protect reactive functional groups, which are structures on amino acids that do not participate in the formation of peptide bonds. These groups are typically acid-labile, meaning they can be removed under mildly acidic conditions without affecting the peptide backbone. Commonly used protecting groups in LPPS include the Boc and Fmoc groups, which protect the amine group on the amino acid.[96]

D. Side-chain deprotection

After the completion of the peptide synthesis, the last peptide molecule is obtained by eliminating the protecting groups from the side chains. This is typically done under mild acidic conditions, such as with TFA. After deprotection, the peptide product can be purified by RP-HPLC.[97]

The chemistry of LPPS involves several key steps, including activation of amino acids, coupling reactions, use of protecting groups, and side-chain deprotection. These steps must be carefully controlled to obtain high yields of pure peptides.

LPPS methodology involves several key steps, including selection of starting materials, preparation of reagents and solvents, synthesis procedure, and purification and characterization of the final product. Each step must be carefully controlled to obtain high yields of pure peptides that can be used for various applications in pharmaceuticals, biotechnology, and chemical research.

Synthesis and characterization of peptides

2.5.6.3 Limitations of LPPS

LPPS offers a wide range of applications, including peptide and protein synthesis, peptide library synthesis, synthesis of problematic amino acids or modified peptides, and cyclic peptide synthesis. These applications make LPPS a valuable tool for drug discovery and development, as well as for reviewing the structure and function of proteins.

Despite the advantages of LPPS in peptide synthesis, several challenges need to be addressed to achieve optimal results. Here are some of the most notable challenges in LPPS:

2.5.6.3.1 Yield optimization

One of the most significant challenges in LPPS is optimizing the yield of the desired peptide. Although LPPS can produce longer peptides compared to SPPS, it is still prone to low yields due to several factors, such as side reactions and incomplete coupling. One way to address this challenge is to optimize the reaction conditions, such as pH, temperature, and coupling reagent concentrations.[98] Additionally, using protected amino acids that are less prone to adverse effects can help increase LPPS output.

2.5.6.3.2 Synthesis of long and complex peptides

Another challenge in LPPS is the production of lengthy and complicated peptides. Although LPPS can produce longer peptides compared to SPPS, it still has limitations in terms of the length and complexity of the peptide. LPPS is particularly challenging to create peptides with numerous disulfide linkages or PTMs, as these can interfere with the coupling reaction and reduce the yield of the desired peptide.[99] To address this challenge, modifications in the coupling reagents, protection groups, and synthetic protocols are continuously being developed to enhance the efficiency of LPPS.

2.5.6.3.3 Purification of peptides from solution

The purification of peptides from solution is another challenge in LPPS. Unlike SPPS, where peptides are attached to a solid support, LPPS produces peptides that are in solution. This makes the purification process more challenging because it entails separating the target peptide from additional contaminants in the solution such as unreacted amino acids, side products, and coupling reagents. One common method of purification in LPPS is the use of RP-HPLC.[99] However, this method is time-consuming and expensive, and can often lead as a result of a low yield of the required peptide. To overcome this challenge, new purification techniques are being developed, such as liquid-liquid extraction and continuous flow systems, to improve the efficiency and yield of LPPS.

Hence, we understand that LPPS has several challenges that need to be addressed to achieve optimal results. These challenges include optimizing the yield of the desired peptide, synthesizing long and complex peptides, and purifying peptides from the solution. Although these challenges can be daunting, advances in the field of LPPS are continuously being made to address these issues, and using this procedure, you can increase the efficiency and yield of the production of peptides.

2.6 HYBRID PEPTIDE SYNTHESIS

The technique of synthesizing peptides using a combination of different methods is known as hybrid peptide synthesis. It involves the integration of both chemical and biological techniques to construct peptides that are hard and difficult to create using conventional methods.[100] The goal of hybrid peptide synthesis is to produce peptides that possess unique structural and functional properties, which can be used in various applications such as drug discovery, vaccine development, and biomaterials engineering.[101]

The importance of hybrid peptide synthesis lies in its ability to expand the scope of peptide chemistry. Traditional peptide synthesis methods are limited in their ability to generate certain types of peptides, such as cyclic peptides or peptides with non-natural amino acids. Hybrid peptide synthesis offers a way to overcome these limitations by using multiple approaches to create peptides with unique properties and functions. Hybrid peptide synthesis also enables the creation of peptides with increased stability, bioactivity, and selectivity, which can be used for a wide range of biomedical applications.[102]

Robert Bruce Merrifield developed SPPS in the mid-20th century, which paved the way for hybrid peptide synthesis. SPPS revolutionized the field of peptide synthesis by allowing for the automated production of peptides on a solid support. However, SPPS was limited by the length of the peptide that could be synthesized, as well as the lack of diversity in the amino acids that could be used.

In the 1990s, Kents colleague's invention of NCL opened up new possibilities for hybrid peptide synthesis. NCL allowed for the synthesis of longer peptides by joining together smaller peptide fragments using a chemoselective reaction.[103] Since then, numerous other methods for hybrid peptide synthesis have been developed, including desulfurization reactions, one-pot synthesis, and computational design.

Hybrid peptide synthesis can be used as an influential tool for expanding the scope of peptide chemistry and creating peptides with unique properties and functions. The integration of different approaches facilitates the synthesis of challenging peptides to create using traditional methods and has numerous applications in fields such as drug discovery, vaccine development, and biomaterials engineering. This history of hybrid peptide production is a testament to the power of innovation and collaboration in advancing scientific knowledge and improving human health.

2.6.1 STRATEGIES FOR HYBRID PEPTIDE SYNTHESIS

Hybrid peptide synthesis is a powerful technique that involves the integration of multiple synthetic approaches to create peptides with unique properties and functions. There are several strategies for hybrid peptide synthesis, each with its advantages and limitations.

Sequential SPPS is a commonly used method for the production of peptides and sequential SPPS where peptide synthesis is performed in a stepwise manner, with each amino acid residue added one to the expanding peptide chain one at a time. Sequential SPPS is an efficient and reliable method for the formation of peptides with lengths of up to 50 amino acids. However, it becomes increasingly difficult to synthesize longer peptides due to the limitations of the solid-phase synthesis process. Sequential SPPS can be combined with other methods, such as NCL or desulfurization reactions, to synthesize longer or more complex peptides.[104]

NCL is a chemoselective procedure inducing the synthesis of longer peptides by joining smaller peptide fragments together. It involves the reaction of a peptide thioester with a peptide containing an N-terminal cysteine residue. The reaction forms a thioester intermediate, which is then hydrolyzed to form a peptide bonde.[103] Because it allows for the assembly of peptide fragments with different functional groups, NCL is a strong approach for the synthesis of longer and more complex peptides. Desulfurization reactions are a type of chemical modification that is used to convert cysteine residues to alanine residues in peptides. This method is particularly useful for the synthesis of cyclic peptides, which often contain cysteine residues.[105] The desulfurization reaction involves the reduction of the sulfur atom in a cysteine residue to form an alanine residue. This modification can increase the stability and bioactivity of the resulting peptide.

One-pot synthesis is a strategy that involves the simultaneous use of multiple synthetic approaches in a single reaction vessel. This approach can be used to synthesize peptides in a more efficient and streamlined manner, as it eliminates the need for multiple purification steps between synthetic stages. One-pot synthesis can be achieved using various methods, such as microwave-assisted synthesis or continuous-flow synthesis.

Other strategies for hybrid peptide synthesis include SPPS with a cleavable linker, which allows for the peptide liberation from the solid support without the need for cleavage using harsh chemicals. Additionally, computational design can be used to predict the structure and properties of hybrid peptides, which can then be synthesized using a combination of different methods.[106]

There are several strategies for hybrid peptide synthesis, each with its advantages and limitations. Sequential SPPS, NCL, desulfurization reactions, one-pot synthesis, and other strategies can be used alone or in combination to synthesize peptides with unique properties and functions. The strategy selected is determined by the specific requirements of the peptide being synthesized, such as length, complexity, and bioactivity. Hybrid peptide synthesis is a potent technique that can be revolutionized in peptide chemistry and has numerous applications in drug discovery, vaccine development, and biomaterials engineering.

2.6.2 CHALLENGES IN HYBRID PEPTIDE SYNTHESIS

Hybrid peptide synthesis is a complex and challenging process that involves the creation of peptides with non-natural amino acids or modifications. While hybrid peptide synthesis has many advantages, there are several challenges that researchers face when attempting to synthesize peptides through this method. We will discuss some of the most difficult issues in hybrid peptide synthesis.

2.6.2.1 Yield and efficiency

Yield and efficiency are significant challenges in hybrid peptide synthesis. Due to the complexity of the synthesis process, yields are often low, and the synthesis can be time-consuming and expensive. One of the reasons for low yields is the high reactivity of some of the synthetic intermediates, which may result in adverse effects and reduced yields.[107] The choice of protecting groups, coupling reagents, and reaction conditions can have a considerable impact on synthesis yield and efficiency.

2.6.2.2 Synthesis of long peptides

The synthesis of long peptides (>50 amino acids) is particularly challenging and time-consuming. Prolonged peptides are challenging to synthesize due to their length, the increased number of reactions required, and the higher likelihood of side reactions. The synthesis of long peptides also requires careful purification and characterization, which can add to the overall time and cost of the synthesis.[107]

2.6.2.3 Formation of regioisomers

The formation of regioisomers is another challenge in hybrid peptide synthesis. Regioisomers are molecules that have the same molecular formula; however, they contrast in terms of atomic connection in the position of functional groups.[108] The formation of regioisomers can occur due to the formation of side products or errors in the synthesis process.[109] Identifying and separating regioisomers can be challenging and time-consuming, resulting in poorer yields and worse purity.

2.6.2.4 Stereochemistry

Stereochemistry is another challenge in hybrid peptide synthesis. Peptides often have several chiral centers, and it is vital to regulator the stereochemistry of the peptide during synthesis. The synthesis of peptides with non-natural amino acids or modifications can lead to increased complexity in the stereochemistry of the peptide.[82] The selection of protecting groups, coupling reagents, and reaction conditions can all affect the stereochemistry of the peptide. To guarantee that the peptide's stereochemistry is correct, these factors must be carefully controlled.

2.6.2.5 Other challenges

Other challenges in hybrid peptide synthesis include the optimization of reaction conditions, purification and characterization of the peptide, and the scalability of the synthesis process. The optimization of reaction conditions can be time-consuming and requires extensive experimentation to achieve optimal yields and efficiency. The peptide purification and characterization also be challenging due to the complexity of the synthesis process, and the scalability of the synthesis process can be difficult due to the need for specialized equipment and expertise.

In conclusion, hybrid peptide synthesis is a complex and challenging process that involves many steps and requires careful attention to detail. Yield and efficiency, synthesis of long peptides, formation of regioisomers, stereochemistry, and other challenges can all impact the success of the synthesis process. Overcoming these challenges requires careful planning, optimization of reaction conditions, and careful purification and characterization of the peptide. Despite these challenges, hybrid peptide synthesis remains a significant tool for the synthesis of peptides with unique features and functions.

2.6.3 Recent advances in hybrid peptide synthesis

Over the past few years, there has been substantial advancement in hybrid peptide synthesis with the development of novel methods and applications. In this section, we will discuss some of the recent advances in hybrid peptide synthesis.

2.6.3.1 Novel methods for efficient synthesis

Efficient synthesis is one of the most difficult issues in hybrid peptide synthesis, and recent advances have focused on developing new methods for improving yields and reducing synthesis time. One such method is the use of microwave-assisted peptide synthesis, which involves the application of microwave radiation to accelerate peptide bond formation.[110] This method has been demonstrated to shorten reaction times and improve yields compared to traditional methods.

Another recent advance is peptide synthesis with flow chemistry, which involves the continuous flow of reagents and reactants through a reactor. Flow chemistry has been shown to reduce reaction times, increase yields, and improve scalability compared to traditional batch synthesis methods.[111]

2.6.3.2 New applications

Hybrid peptide synthesis has also seen new applications in areas including drug discovery, bioconjugation, and material science. One recent application is the advance of hybrid peptides for targeted drug delivery. Hybrid peptides can be engineered to deliver therapeutic substances into particular cells or tissues with high specificity and efficiency.[112]

Another application is the use of hybrid peptides for bioconjugation, which involves the attachment of biomolecules to nonbiological molecules. Hybrid peptides can be used as linkers or spacers for the attachment of various biomolecules, including proteins, nucleic acids, and small molecules.[113]

In material science, hybrid peptides are used as blocks for the synthesis of novel materials with unique properties, such as hydrogels and nanomaterials.[114] These materials have applications in tissue engineering- drug delivery and other areas.

2.6.3.3 Computational design of hybrid peptides
Computational design is another area of recent progress in hybrid peptide synthesis. Computational methods can be used to design hybrid peptides with specific properties and functions, such as increased stability, affinity, or enzymatic activity.[103] These methods can also be used to predict the folding and conformation of hybrid peptides, which is important for their biological activity.

2.6.3.4 Other advances
Other recent advances in hybrid peptide synthesis include the development of new protecting groups and coupling reagents, as well as the use of novel amino acids and modifications. For example, the development of thioamide-containing amino acids has led to the synthesis of more stable and protease-resistant peptides.[115]

Hybrid peptide production has made significant progress in recent years, while these advances have the potential to revolutionize the field of peptide synthesis and lead to the development of new and innovative products with unique properties and functions.

2.7 PURIFICATION AND CHARACTERIZATION OF PEPTIDES

Due to their diverse biological activities including signal transduction, enzyme regulation, and immune response, peptides have become attractive targets for drug discovery and development. However, the purification and characterization of peptides can be difficult due to their scarcity and structural complexity.

Peptide purification involves the separation of the desired peptide from a complex mixture of proteins, peptides, and other impurities. Various chromatographic and electrophoretic techniques are commonly used for peptide purification.[116] Once purified, the characterization of peptides is necessary to understand their properties, such as their amino acid sequence, structural conformation, and bioactivity.

Accurate peptide purification and characterization are essential for the development of peptide-based therapeutics, as even minor variations in the peptide structure or purity can affect its biological activity and safety. Therefore, the development of efficient and reliable methods for peptide purification and characterization is of great importance for advancing peptide-based drug discovery and development.

Peptides are short sequences of amino acids that serve important roles in many biological processes. However, the isolation and purification of peptides from complex mixtures can be due to their scarcity, structural variety, and susceptibility to deterioration.

Peptides can be obtained from various sources, including natural sources such as proteins, tissues, and fluids, as well as synthetic sources such as SPPS. Natural sources of peptides are further classified as endogenous (made by the body) and exogenous (generated outside the body or obtained from external sources). Endogenous peptides are commonly found in tissues, blood, urine, and other bodily fluids, while exogenous peptides are obtained from plants, animals, and microorganisms.[117]

Initial sample preparation: Before the purification process begins, the initial sample must be prepared to remove unwanted materials and concentrate the target peptide. The initial sample preparation can vary depending on the source and type of peptide, but common methods include acid or base treatment, lyophilization, or solid-phase extraction.

Chromatographic techniques are widely used for the purification of peptides due to their facility to distinguish compounds based on their physicochemical properties. The most commonly used chromatographic techniques for peptide purification include ion exchange chromatography, size exclusion chromatography, and RP-HPLC.[116]

Ion exchange chromatography separates peptides based on their charge, with positively charged peptides binding to negatively charged resin and vice versa. Size exclusion chromatography separates peptides based on their size, with larger peptides eluting first from the column. RP-HPLC peptides are classified based on their hydrophobicity, with hydrophobic peptides interacting with the stationary phase.[118]

In addition to chromatography, other purification methods can be used for the isolation of peptides. These methods include HPLC, fast protein liquid chromatography (FPLC),[119] and electrophoresis. HPLC is a highly efficient and precise chromatographic technique that utilizes high-pressure pumps and small particle sizes for improved resolution. FPLC is a more versatile version of HPLC that allows for the purification of larger molecules. Electrophoresis, on the other hand, separates peptides based on their charge and size and is useful for separating peptides with similar properties.[120]

Yield determination: After the peptide purification process is complete, the yield must be determined to ensure the purity and efficiency of the purification process. The yield is typically quantified by measuring the amount of peptide in the purified sample using spectrophotometry, amino acid analysis, or a bioassay.

Thus, we understand that purification of peptides is an essential step in peptide research and drug development. Various methods can be used to isolate and purify peptides, including chromatographic techniques, electrophoresis, and other purification methods. The method of filtration adopted will be determined by the properties of the peptide and the desired level of purity. Accurate yield determination is necessary to evaluate the efficiency of the purification process and ensure the purity of the final peptide product.

Peptide purification and characterization are critical steps in peptide research since it is crucial in the development of peptide-based medicines. Accurate purification and characterization of peptides ensure the purity, homogeneity, and bioactivity of the final product, which are essential for drug discovery and development.

The improvement of efficient and reliable methods for peptide purification and characterization has led to the discovery of several promising peptide-based drugs. For example, the peptide hormone insulin is a frequently used therapeutic medication for diabetes, and the peptide-based drug enfuvirtide is used for the treatment of human immunodeficiency virus (HIV).[121] In addition, several peptide-based drugs are currently in clinical trials for the treatment of cancer, infectious diseases, and other medical conditions.

The future of peptide research is promising, with the creation of novel peptide synthesis technologies, purification, and characterization. For example, advances in SPPS have led to the rapid and efficient production of peptides, while new purification techniques, such as preparative HPLC and membrane-based separation,[21] have improved the efficiency and accuracy of peptide purification.

Furthermore, the development of new techniques for peptide characterization, such as hydrogen-deuterium exchange mass spectrometry, native mass spectrometry, and cryogenic electron microscopy, has enabled the determination of the structural and functional properties of peptides at high resolution.

Hence, we understand that peptide purification and characterization are essential for the development of peptide-based therapeutics. The continued development of new methods and techniques for peptide purification and characterization will further contribute to the advancement of peptide research and the discovery of novel peptide-based medications for the treatment of various medical conditions.

2.8 MASS SPECTROMETRY AND NMR SPECTROSCOPY

Mass spectrometry and NMR spectroscopy are two dominant analytical techniques that are extensively used in a variety of fields of science, including chemistry, biology, and materials science. Both techniques provide detailed information about the structure, composition, and properties of molecules and materials.

2.8.1 Mass Spectrometry

The mass-to-charge ratio (m/z) of ions in a sample can be determined using mass spectrometry.[122] It entails ionizing a sample to produce charged particles, which are subsequently separated using an electric and/or magnetic field based on their mass-to-charge ratio. The resulting spectrum contains information on the molecular weight and structure of the substance sample.[123]

There are several ionization methods used in mass spectrometry, including electron ionization (EI), electrospray ionization (ESI), and matrix-assisted laser desorption/ionization (MALDI).[122] EI is typically used for small, volatile compounds, while ESI and MALDI are used for larger, nonvolatile compounds.

Synthesis and characterization of peptides 41

In addition to providing information on the sample's molecular weight and the ionization of the structure, mass spectrometry can also be used to identify unknown compounds and quantify the amount of a particular compound in a sample. It is commonly utilized in proteomics, metabolomics, and drug discovery.[124]

2.8.2 NMR Spectroscopy

NMR spectroscopy is a technique used to investigate the structure and dynamics of molecules. It is based on the magnetic properties of certain atomic nuclei, such as hydrogen, carbon, and nitrogen. When placed in a strong magnetic field, these nuclei absorb energy at specific frequencies, which can be detected and used to obtain information about the molecule.

NMR spectroscopy could identify the number and kind of atoms in a molecule, as well as the arrangement in space.[125] It is beneficial for determining the structure of organic compounds, such as proteins and nucleic acids.

There are several types of NMR spectroscopy, including proton NMR, carbon-13 NMR, and heteronuclear NMR.[126] Proton NMR is the most commonly used, as it provides information on the hydrogen atoms in a molecule. Carbon-13 NMR is used to study the carbon atoms in a molecule, while heteronuclear NMR is used to investigate the connections of various types of nuclei in a molecule. NMR spectroscopy is widely employed in many disciplines, including chemistry, biochemistry, and materials research, and has many applications in drug discovery, metabolomics, and structural biology.[127]

These two powerful analytical techniques give useful information about the structure, composition, and characteristics of molecules and materials. They are widely used in various fields of science and have many important applications in research and industry.

2.9 OTHER METHODS FOR PEPTIDE CHARACTERIZATION

Some of the other methods used for peptide characterization include:

1. **X-ray crystallography**: This is a method for determining the three-dimensional structure of molecules, including peptides and proteins. It involves the crystallization of the molecule of interest, followed by the use of X-rays to determine the positions of the atoms in the crystal lattice. X-ray crystallography provides high-resolution structural data, facilitating the establishment of precise locations of individual atoms within a molecule.
2. **CD spectroscopy**: CD spectroscopy is a technique used to study the secondary structure of peptides and proteins. It involves the measurement of a molecule's asymmetrical absorption of left- and right-circularly polarized light. The resulting spectrum provides data based on the type and amount of secondary structure present in the molecule, including alpha-helices, beta-sheets, and random coils.

3. **Fourier transform infrared (FTIR) spectroscopy**: This is an instrument used to study the vibrational modes of molecules, including peptides and proteins. It comprises an analysis of a sample's absorption or transmission of infrared radiation. The resulting spectrum provides information on the functional groups present in the molecule, including amide bonds, which are characteristic features of peptides and proteins.
4. **HPLC**: This is helpful in the separation and purification of peptides and proteins. It comprises the procedure of a stationary phase, such as a column packed with a resin, and a mobile phase, such as a buffer solution. After injecting the sample into the column, the components divide depending on their interactions with the stationary and mobile phases. HPLC can be used for the purification of peptides and proteins, as well as for the separation and identification of different many components in a blend.
5. **Edman degradation**: Edman degradation is a method used with chemicals for the sequencing of peptides. It involves the selective removal of the N-terminal amino acid from a peptide, which is then identified by mass spectrometry or other analytical techniques. Edman degradation can be used for the sequencing of peptides up to 50–60 amino acids in length.

In conclusion, there are several other methods used for peptide characterization in addition to mass spectrometry and NMR spectroscopy. These methods provide complementary and can be used in conjunction with mass spectrometry to provide information on the structure, content, and characteristics of peptides and proteins, and NMR spectroscopy to provide a more complete characterization of these molecules.

2.10 RECENT ADVANCES IN PEPTIDE SYNTHESIS AND CHARACTERIZATION

Peptides are small chains of amino acids that serve critical roles in a variety of biological processes such as cell signaling, enzyme catalysis, and immunological function. The synthesis and characterization of peptides are essential for understanding their biological function and for the development of peptide-based therapeutics. New advances in peptide synthesis and characterization have resulted in significant gains in efficiency, specificity, and stability with a diversity of peptide synthesis and characterization methods.

2.10.1 PEPTIDE SYNTHESIS

The traditional method of peptide synthesis involves sequential amino acid incorporation to a developing peptide chain, using a protecting group strategy to prevent unwanted side reactions. While this method is still widely used, recent advances have focused on improving the efficiency and specificity of peptide synthesis.

One major advance has been the development of new coupling reagents and strategies that allow for faster and more efficient peptide synthesis. For example, the use of microwave irradiation has been shown to significantly decrease the time required for peptide coupling reactions, while also increasing the ultimate product's quantity and purity. Other advances in coupling reagents and strategies have focused on reducing side reactions and increasing the specificity of peptide synthesis.

Another major change in peptide synthesis is the development of new SPPS techniques. SPPS involves peptide immobilization on a solid support, allowing for the efficient and selective addition of amino acids to the developing peptide chain. Recent advances in SPPS have focused on improving the efficiency and specificity of the technique, as well as on expanding the range of amino acids and modifications that can be incorporated into peptides.

2.10.2 Peptide characterization

The characterization of peptides is essential for understanding their structure and function, including the development of therapeutic-based peptides. Recent advances in peptide characterization have focused on improving the sensitivity, resolution, and speed of analytical techniques.

One major advance has been the creation of new mass spectrometry techniques for peptide analysis. This procedure allows for the rapid and sensitive identification and quantification of peptides, as well as for the determination of their sequence and modifications. Recent advances in mass spectrometry have focused on improving the resolution and sensitivity of the technique, as well as on developing new fragmentation strategies that allow for more comprehensive peptide analysis.

Another major improvement in peptide characterization is the development of new NMR spectroscopy techniques. NMR spectroscopy allows for the determination of the three-dimensional structure of peptides, as well as for the characterization of their interactions with other molecules. Recent advances in NMR spectroscopy have focused on improving the resolution and sensitivity of the technique, as well as on developing novel techniques for studying bigger peptides and protein complexes.

In conclusion, recent advances in peptide synthesis and characterization have led to significant improvements in the efficiency, specificity, and diversity of peptide synthesis and characterization methods. These advances have important implications for the study of biological functions, and the development of peptide-based medicines is likely to drive peptide research innovation in the future years.

2.11 PRACTICAL QUESTIONS

1. What is the process of peptide synthesis, and what are the key methods used to create peptides with different levels of complexity and lengths?

2. How is the purity of synthesized peptides assessed, and what are the major purification techniques employed to obtain high-quality peptides for characterization?
3. How do techniques such as mass spectrometry, NMR, and chromatography contribute to identifying and confirming the structure of peptides?
4. In peptide design and synthesis, what are the common strategies to enhance peptide stability, bioactivity, and specificity?
5. What are the applications of synthesized peptides in biomedical research, pharmaceuticals, and biotechnology?

REFERENCES

1. Bulaj, G.; Olivera, B. M., Folding of conotoxins: Formation of the native disulfide bridges during chemical synthesis and biosynthesis of Conus peptides. *Antioxidants & Redox Signaling* **2008**, 10 (1), 141–156.
2. Sit, C. S.; Yoganathan, S.; Vederas, J. C., Biosynthesis of aminovinyl-cysteine-containing peptides and its application in the production of potential drug candidates. *Accounts of Chemical Research* **2011**, 44 (4), 261–268.
3. Kachala, V. V.; Khemchyan, L. L. v.; Kashin, A. S.; Orlov, N.; Grachev, A. A.; Zalesskiy, S.; Ananikov, V. P., Target-oriented analysis of gaseous, liquid and solid chemical systems by mass spectrometry, nuclear magnetic resonance spectroscopy and electron microscopy. *Russian Chemical Reviews* **2013**, 82 (7), 648.
4. Weissbach, H., *Molecular mechanisms of protein biosynthesis*. Elsevier: 2012.
5. Miller Jr, O.; Hamkalo, B. A., Visualization of RNA synthesis on chromosomes. *International Review of Cytology* **1972**, 33, 1–25.
6. Alberts, B.; Johnson, A.; Lewis, J.; Raff, M.; Roberts, K.; Walter, P., From DNA to RNA. In *Molecular biology of the cell*. 4th edition, Garland Science: 2002.
7. Minchin, S.; Lodge, J., Understanding biochemistry: Structure and function of nucleic acids. *Essays in Biochemistry* **2019**, 63 (4), 433–456.
8. Clancy, S.; Brown, W., Translation: DNA up mRNA to protein. *Nature Education* **2008**, 1 (1), 101.
9. Sanvictores, T.; Farci, F., *Biochemistry, primary protein structure*. StatPearls Publishing, 2020.
10. Clancy, S.; Brownish, W., *Where translation occurs*.
11. Drake, E. J.; Miller, B. R.; Shi, C.; Tarrasch, J. T.; Sundlov, J. A.; Leigh Allen, C.; Skiniotis, G.; Aldrich, C. C.; Gulick, A. M., Structures of two distinct conformations of holo-non-ribosomal peptide synthetases. *Nature* **2016**, 529 (7585), 235–238.
12. Tajbakhsh, M.; Karimi, A.; Fallah, F.; Akhavan, M., Overview of ribosomal and non-ribosomal antimicrobial peptides produced by Gram positive bacteria. *Cellular and Molecular Biology* **2017**, 63 (10), 20–32.
13. Dinman, J. D., Mechanisms and implications of programmed translational frameshifting. *Wiley Interdisciplinary Reviews: RNA* **2012**, 3 (5), 661–673.
14. Payne, J. A.; Schoppet, M.; Hansen, M. H.; Cryle, M. J., Diversity of nature's assembly lines–recent discoveries in non-ribosomal peptide synthesis. *Molecular BioSystems* **2017**, 13 (1), 9–22.
15. Bozhüyük, K. A.; Fleischhacker, F.; Linck, A.; Wesche, F.; Tietze, A.; Niesert, C.-P.; Bode, H. B., De novo design and engineering of non-ribosomal peptide synthetases. *Nature Chemistry* **2018**, 10 (3), 275–281.

16. Eisfeld, K., Non-ribosomal peptide synthetases of fungi. *Physiology and Genetics: Selected Basic and Applied Aspects* 2009, 15, 305–330.
17. Holland, A.; Kinnear, S., Interpreting the possible ecological role (s) of cyanotoxins: Compounds for competitive advantage and/or physiological aide? *Marine Drugs* **2013**, *11* (7), 2239–2258.
18. Muramatsu, W.; Manthena, C.; Nakashima, E.; Yamamoto, H., Peptide bond-forming reaction via amino acid silyl esters: New catalytic reactivity of an aminosilane. *ACS Catalysis* **2020**, 10 (16), 9594–9603.
19. Stojanoski, K.; Zdravkovski, Z., On the formation of peptide bonds. *Journal of Chemical Education* **1993**, 70 (2), 134.
20. Avan, I.; Hall, C. D.; Katritzky, A. R., Peptidomimetics via modifications of amino acids and peptide bonds. *Chemical Society Reviews* 2014, 43 (10), 3575–3594.
21. Behrendt, R.; White, P.; Offer, J., Advances in Fmoc solid-phase peptide synthesis. *Journal of Peptide Science* **2016**, 22 (1), 4–27.
22. Carpino, L. A.; Ghassemi, S.; Ionescu, D.; Ismail, M.; Sadat-Aalaee, D.; Truran, G. A.; Mansour, E.; Siwruk, G. A.; Eynon, J. S.; Morgan, B., Rapid, continuous solution-phase peptide synthesis: Application to peptides of pharmaceutical interest. *Organic Process Research & Development* **2003**, 7 (1), 28–37.
23. Mahindra, A.; Sharma, K. K.; Jain, R., Rapid microwave-assisted solution-phase peptide synthesis. *Tetrahedron Letters* **2012**, 53 (51), 6931–6935.
24. Choi, S.-H.; Jeong, W.-J.; Choi, S.-J.; Lim, Y.-B., Highly efficient and fast pre-activation cyclization of the long peptide: Succinimidyl ester-amine reaction revisited. *Bioorganic & Medicinal Chemistry Letters* **2015**, 25 (22), 5335–5338.
25. Simon, M. D.; Heider, P. L.; Adamo, A.; Vinogradov, A. A.; Mong, S. K.; Li, X.; Berger, T.; Policarpo, R. L.; Zhang, C.; Zou, Y., Rapid flow-based peptide synthesis. *ChemBioChem* **2014**, 15 (5), 713–720.
26. Seibert, C.; Sakmar, T. P., Toward a framework for sulfoproteomics: Synthesis and characterization of sulfotyrosine-containing peptides. *Peptide Science* **2008**, 90 (3), 459–477.
27. Merrifield, R. B., Solid phase peptide synthesis. I. The synthesis of a tetrapeptide. *Journal of the American Chemical Society* **1963**, 85 (14), 2149–2154.
28. Junk, G.; Svec, H., The mass spectra of the α-amino acids. *Journal of the American Chemical Society* **1963**, 85 (7), 839–845.
29. Warner, J. R.; Knopf, P. M.; Rich, A., A multiple ribosomal structure in protein synthesis. *Proceedings of the National Academy of Sciences* **1963**, 49 (1), 122–129.
30. Fields, G. B.; Noble, R. L., Solid phase peptide synthesis utilizing 9-fluorenylmethoxycarbonyl amino acids. *International Journal of Peptide and Protein Research* **1990**, 35 (3), 161–214.
31. Krchňák, V.; Holladay, M. W., Solid phase heterocyclic chemistry. *Chemical Reviews* **2002**, 102 (1), 61–92.
32. Paypanova, T.; Hristova, T., Synthesis of oligopeptides of defined fragment composition. *Journal of IMAB–Annual Proceeding Scientific Papers* **2011**, 17 (1), 127–129.
33. Santini, R.; Griffith, M. C.; Qi, M., A measure of solvent effects on swelling of resins for solid phase organic synthesis. *Tetrahedron Letters* **1998**, 39 (49), 8951–8954.
34. Barlos, K.; Chatzi, O.; Gatos, D.; Stavropoulos, G., 2-Chlorotrityl chloride resin. Studies on anchoring of Fmoc-amino acids and peptide cleavage. *International Journal of Peptide and Protein Research* **1991**, 37 (6), 513–520.
35. Hansen, J.; Diness, F.; Meldal, M., C-Terminally modified peptides via cleavage of the HMBA linker by O-, N- or S-nucleophiles. *Organic & Biomolecular Chemistry* **2016**, 14 (12), 3238–3245.

36. Pedersen, S. L.; Jensen, K. J., Peptide release, side-chain deprotection, work-up, and isolation. *Methods in Molecular Biology (Clifton, N.J.)* **2013**, 1047, 43–63.
37. Sieber, P., A new acid-labile anchor group for the solid-phase synthesis of C-terminal peptide amides by the Fmoc method. *Tetrahedron Letters* **1987**, 28 (19), 2107–2110.
38. Sherrington, D. C., Preparation, structure and morphology of polymer supports. *Chemical Communications* **1998**, (21), 2275–2286.
39. Quarrell, R.; Claridge, T. D. W.; Weaver, G. W.; Lowe, G., Structure and properties of TentaGel resin beads: Implications for combinatorial library chemistry. *Molecular Diversity* **1996**, *1* (4), 223–232.
40. Kempe, M.; Barany, G., CLEAR: A novel family of highly cross-linked polymeric supports for solid-phase peptide synthesis1,2. *Journal of the American Chemical Society* **1996**, 118 (30), 7083–7093.
41. Crich, D.; Sana, K., Solid-phase synthesis of peptidyl thioacids employing a 9-fluorenylmethyl thioester-based linker in conjunction with Boc chemistry. *The Journal of Organic Chemistry* 2009, 74 (19), 7383–7388.
42. Sun, Y.; Frenkel-Pinter, M.; Liotta, C. L.; Grover, M. A., The pH dependent mechanisms of non-enzymatic peptide bond cleavage reactions. Physical Chemistry Chemical Physics 2020, 22 (1), 107–113.
43. Albericio, F., Orthogonal protecting groups for Nα-amino and C-terminal carboxyl functions in solid-phase peptide synthesis. *Peptide Science* **2000**, 55 (2), 123–139.
44. Masui, Y.; Chino, N.; Sakakibara, S., The modification of Tryptophyl residues during the acidolytic cleavage of Boc-groups. I. Studies with Boc-Tryptophan. *Bulletin of the Chemical Society of Japan* **1980**, 53 (2), 464–468.
45. Carpino, L. A., The 9-fluorenylmethyloxycarbonyl family of base-sensitive amino-protecting groups. *Accounts of Chemical Research* **1987**, 20 (11), 401–407.
46. Kessler, H.; Siegmeier, R., 9-Fluorenylmethyl esters as carboxyl protecting group. *Tetrahedron Letters* **1983**, 24 (3), 281–282.
47. Gundala, C.; Tantry, S. J.; Naik, S. A.; Sureshbabu, V. V., Synthesis of 1, 1-Dioxobenzo [b] thiophene-2-ylmethyloxycarbonyl (Bsmoc) protected N-Methyl amino acids by reduction of Bsmoc-5-Oxazolidinones and their use in peptide synthesis. *Protein and Peptide Letters* 2009, 16 (2), 105–111.
48. Carpino, L. A.; Philbin, M.; Ismail, M.; Truran, G. A.; Mansour, E. M. E.; Iguchi, S.; Ionescu, D.; El-Faham, A.; Riemer, C.; Warrass, R.; Weiss, M. S., New family of base - and nucleophile-sensitive amino-protecting groups. A Michael-acceptor-based deblocking process. Practical utilization of the 1,1-Dioxobenzo[b]thiophene-2-ylmethyloxycarbonyl (Bsmoc) group. *Journal of the American Chemical Society* **1997**, *119* (41), 9915–9916.
49. Carpino, L. A.; Abdel-Maksoud, A. A.; Ionescu, D.; Mansour, E.; Zewail, M. A., 1, 1-dioxonaphtho [1, 2–b] thiophene-2-methyloxycarbonyl (α-Nsmoc) and 3, 3-dioxonaphtho [2, 1–b] thiophene-2-methyloxycarbonyl (β-Nsmoc) aminoprotecting groups. *The Journal of Organic Chemistry* 2007, 72 (5), 1729–1736.
50. Díaz-Mochón, J. J.; Bialy, L.; Bradley, M., Full orthogonality between Dde and Fmoc: The direct synthesis of PNA– peptide conjugates. *Organic Letters* **2004**, 6 (7), 1127–1129.
51. Debenham, J. S.; Debenham, S. D.; Fraser-Reid, B., N-Tetrachlorophthaloyl (TCP) for ready protection/deprotection of amino sugar glycosides. *Bioorganic & Medicinal Chemistry* **1996**, 4 (11), 1909–1918.
52. Cros, E.; Planas, M.; Barany, G.; Bardají, E., N-Tetrachlorophthaloyl (TCP) protection for solid-phase peptide synthesis. *European Journal of Organic Chemistry* 2004, *2004* (17), 3633–3642.

53. Hojo, K.; Maeda, M.; Kawasaki, K., A new water-soluble N-protecting group, 2-[phenyl (methyl) sulfonio] ethyloxycarbonyl tetrafluoroborate, and its application to solid phase peptide synthesis in water. *Journal of Peptide Science: An Official Publication of the European Peptide Society* **2001**, 7 (12), 615–618.
54. Weygand, F.; Frauendorfer, E., Reductive elimination of the N-trifluoroacetyl and N-trichloroacetyl group by sodium boron hydride and applications in peptide chemistry. *Chemische Berichte* **1970**, 103 (8), 2437–2449.
55. Bellamy, A. J.; MacCuish, A.; Golding, P.; Mahon, M. F., The use of Trifluoroacetyl as an N-and O-protecting group during the synthesis of energetic compounds containing Nitramine and/or Nitrate Ester groups. *Propellants, Explosives, Pyrotechnics: An International Journal Dealing with Scientific and Technological Aspects of Energetic Materials* **2007**, 32 (1), 20–31.
56. Behloul, C.; Guijarro, D.; Yus, M., Detritylation of N-tritylamines via a naphthalene-catalyzed lithiation process. *Synthesis* **2004**, *2004* (8), 1274–1280.
57. Nottingham, M.; Bethel, C. R.; Pagadala, S. R. R.; Harry, E.; Pinto, A.; Lemons, Z. A.; Drawz, S. M.; Van Den Akker, F.; Carey, P. R.; Bonomo, R. A., Modifications of the C6-substituent of penicillin sulfones with the goal of improving inhibitor recognition and efficacy. *Bioorganic & Medicinal Chemistry Letters* **2011**, 21 (1), 387–393.
58. Zaramella, S.; Yeheskiely, E.; Strömberg, R., A method for solid-phase synthesis of oligonucleotide 5'-peptide-conjugates using acid-labile α-amino protections. *Journal of the American Chemical Society* **2004**, 126 (43), 14029–14035.
59. Barzilay, I.; Lapidot, Y., The use of o-nitrophenylsulfenyl group as amino protecting group in the synthesis of phosphatidylethanolamine. Chemistry and Physics of Lipids 1971, 7 (1–2), 93–97.
60. Zervas, L.; Borovas, D.; Gazis, E., New methods in peptide synthesis. I. Tritylsulfenyl and o-nitrophenylsulfenyl groups as N-protecting groups. *Journal of the American Chemical Society* **1963**, 85 (22), 3660–3666.
61. Sarkar, A.; Roy, S. R.; Parikh, N.; Chakraborti, A. K., Nonsolvent application of ionic liquids: Organo-catalysis by 1-alkyl-3-methylimidazolium cation based room-temperature ionic liquids for chemoselective N-tert-butyloxycarbonylation of amines and the influence of the C-2 hydrogen on catalytic efficiency. *The Journal of Organic Chemistry* 2011, 76 (17), 7132–7140.
62. McKay, F. C.; Albertson, N. F., New amine-masking groups for peptide synthesis. *Journal of the American Chemical Society* **1957**, 79 (17), 4686–4690.
63. Englund, E. A.; Gopi, H. N.; Appella, D. H., An efficient synthesis of a probe for protein function: 2, 3-diaminopropionic acid with orthogonal protecting groups. *Organic Letters* **2004**, 6 (2), 213–215.
64. Kiso, Y.; Ukawa, K.; Akita, T., Efficient removal of N-benzyloxycarbonyl group by a 'push–pull' mechanism using thioanisole–trifluoroacetic acid, exemplified by a synthesis of Met-enkephalin. *Journal of the Chemical Society, Chemical Communications* **1980**, (3), 101–102.
65. Perron, V.; Abbott, S.; Moreau, N.; Lee, D.; Penney, C.; Zacharie, B., A method for the selective protection of aromatic amines in the presence of aliphatic amines. *Synthesis* **2009**, *2009* (02), 283–289.
66. Bregant, S.; Tabor, A. B., Orthogonally protected lanthionines: Synthesis and use for the solid-phase synthesis of an analogue of nisin ring C. *The Journal of Organic Chemistry* **2005**, 70 (7), 2430–2438.
67. Martinez, J.; Laur, J.; Castro, B., Carboxamidomethyl esters (CAM esters) as carboxyl protecting groups. *Tetrahedron Letters* **1983**, 24 (47), 5219–5222.

68. Di Gioia, M. L.; Leggio, A.; Le Pera, A.; Liguori, A.; Perri, F.; Siciliano, C., Alternative and chemoselective deprotection of the α-amino and carboxy functions of N-Fmoc-Amino Acid and N-Fmoc-Dipeptide Methyl Esters by modulation of the molar ratio in the AlCl3/N, N-Dimethylaniline reagent system. *European Journal of Organic Chemistry* 2004, 2004 (21), 4437–4441.
69. Martinez, J.; Laur, J.; Castro, B., On the use of carboxamidomethyl esters (Cam esters) in the synthesis of model peptides. Scope and limitations. *Tetrahedron* **1985**, 41 (4), 739–743.
70. Chen, R.; Tolbert, T. J., On-resin convergent synthesis of a glycopeptide from HIV gp120 containing a high mannose type N-linked oligosaccharide. *Bioconjugation Protocols: Strategies and Methods* 2011, 751, 343–355.
71. Isidro-Llobet, A.; Alvarez, M.; Albericio, F., Amino acid-protecting groups. *Chemical Reviews* **2009**, 109 (6), 2455–2504.
72. Kaul, R.; Brouillette, Y.; Sajjadi, Z.; Hansford, K. A.; Lubell, W. D., Selective tert-butyl ester deprotection in the presence of acid labile protecting groups with use of ZnBr2. *The Journal of Organic Chemistry* **2004**, 69 (18), 6131–6133.
73. Shi, H.; Nie, K.; Dong, B.; Chao, L.; Gao, F.; Ma, M.; Long, M.; Liu, Z., Mixing enhancement via a serpentine micromixer for real-time activation of carboxyl. *Chemical Engineering Journal* **2020**, 392, 123642.
74. Han, S.-Y.; Kim, Y.-A., Recent development of peptide coupling reagents in organic synthesis. *Tetrahedron* **2004**, 60 (11), 2447–2468.
75. Bruckdorfer, T.; Marder, O.; Albericio, F., From production of peptides in milligram amounts for research to multi-tons quantities for drugs of the future. *Current Pharmaceutical Biotechnology* **2004**, 5 (1), 29–43.
76. Tam, J. P.; Heath, W. F.; Merrifield, R., SN 1 and SN 2 mechanisms for the deprotection of synthetic peptides by hydrogen fluoride: Studies to minimize the tyrosine alkylation side reaction. *International Journal of Peptide and Protein Research* **1983**, 21 (1), 57–65.
77. Sampson, W. R.; Patsiouras, H.; Ede, N. J., The synthesis of 'difficult'peptides using 2-hydroxy-4-methoxybenzyl or pseudoproline amino acid building blocks: A comparative study. *Journal of Peptide Science: An Official Publication of the European Peptide Society* **1999**, 5 (9), 403–409.
78. Beaufils, D.; Danger, G.; Boiteau, L.; Rossi, J.-C.; Pascal, R., Diastereoselectivity in prebiotically relevant 5 (4 H)-oxazolone-mediated peptide couplings. *Chemical Communications* 2014, 50 (23), 3100–3102.
79. Schelhaas, M.; Waldmann, H., Protecting group strategies in organic synthesis. *Angewandte Chemie International Edition in English* **1996**, 35 (18), 2056–2083.
80. Schäfer, O.; Barz, M., Of thiols and disulfides: Methods for chemoselective formation of asymmetric disulfides in synthetic peptides and polymers. *Chemistry–A European Journal* **2018**, 24 (47), 12131–12142.
81. David, R.; Richter, M. P.; Beck-Sickinger, A. G., Expressed protein ligation: Method and applications. *European Journal of Biochemistry* **2004**, 271 (4), 663–677.
82. Gentilucci, L.; De Marco, R.; Cerisoli, L., Chemical modifications designed to improve peptide stability: Incorporation of non-natural amino acids, pseudo-peptide bonds, and cyclization. *Current Pharmaceutical Design* 2010, 16 (28), 3185–3203.
83. Conibear, A. C.; Watson, E. E.; Payne, R. J.; Becker, C. F., Native chemical ligation in protein synthesis and semi-synthesis. *Chemical Society Reviews* **2018**, 47 (24), 9046–9068.
84. Gates, Z. P.; Hartrampf, N., Flow-based SPPS for protein synthesis: A perspective. *Peptide Science* **2020**, *112* (6), e24198.

85. Kent, S. B., Chemical synthesis of peptides and proteins. *Annual Review of Biochemistry* **1988**, 57 (1), 957–989.
86. Palasek, S. A.; Cox, Z. J.; Collins, J. M., Limiting racemization and aspartimide formation in microwave-enhanced Fmoc solid phase peptide synthesis. *Journal of Peptide Science: An Official Publication of the European Peptide Society* **2007**, 13 (3), 143–148.
87. Cuatrecasas, P.; Anfinsen, C. B., [31] Affinity chromatography. *Methods in Enzymology* **1971**, 22, 345–378.
88. Lawrenson, S.; North, M.; Peigneguy, F.; Routledge, A., Greener solvents for solid-phase synthesis. Green Chemistry 2017, 19 (4), 952–962.
89. Bayer, E.; Mutter, M., Liquid phase synthesis of peptides. *Nature* **1972**, 237 (5357), 512–513.
90. Bayer, E.; Mutter, M.; Uhmann, R.; Polster, J.; Mauser, H., Kinetic studies of the liquid phase peptide synthesis. *Journal of the American Chemical Society* **1974**, 96 (23), 7333–7336.
91. Han, H.; Wolfe, M. M.; Brenner, S.; Janda, K. D., Liquid-phase combinatorial synthesis. *Proceedings of the National Academy of Sciences* **1995**, 92 (14), 6419–6423.
92. Jaradat, D. s. M., Thirteen decades of peptide synthesis: Key developments in solid phase peptide synthesis and amide bond formation utilized in peptide ligation. *Amino Acids* **2018**, 50 (1), 39–68.
93. Takahashi, D.; Yano, T.; Fukui, T., Novel diphenylmethyl-derived amide protecting group for efficient liquid-phase peptide synthesis: AJIPHASE. *Organic Letters* **2012**, 14 (17), 4514–4517.
94. Kovacs, J.; Kisfaludy, L.; Ceprini, M. Q., On the optical purity of peptide active esters prepared by N,N′-Dicyclohexylcarbodiimide and "Complexes" of N,N′-Dicyclohexylcarbodiimide-Pentachlorophenol and N,N′-Dicyclohexylcarbodiimide-Pentafluorophenol. *Journal of the American Chemical Society* **1967**, 89 (1), 183–184.
95. El-Faham, A.; Albericio, F., Peptide coupling reagents, more than a letter soup. *Chemical Reviews* **2011**, 111 (11), 6557–6602.
96. Ten Brummelhuis, N.; Wilke, P.; Börner, H. G., Peptide synthesis and beyond the use of sequence-defined segments for materials science. *Sequence-Controlled Polymers,* Macromolecular Rapid Communications, **2018**, 38 (24),117–158.
97. Todd, S., *Designing surfaces to direct cell behaviour.* The University of Manchester: 2007.
98. Christopher, L. P.; Kumar, H.; Zambare, V. P., Enzymatic biodiesel: Challenges and opportunities. *Applied Energy* 2014, 119, 497–520.
99. Gauthier, M. A.; Klok, H.-A., Peptide/protein–polymer conjugates: Synthetic strategies and design concepts. *Chemical Communications* **2008**, (23), 2591–2611.
100. Sieber, S. A.; Marahiel, M. A., Molecular mechanisms underlying nonribosomal peptide synthesis: Approaches to new antibiotics. *Chemical Reviews* **2005**, 105 (2), 715–738.
101. Löwik, D. W.; Ayres, L.; Smeenk, J. M.; Van Hest, J. C., Synthesis of bio-inspired hybrid polymers using peptide synthesis and protein engineering. *Peptide Hybrid Polymers* 2006, 202, 19–52.
102. Wang, Y.; Xia, K.; Wang, L.; Wu, M.; Sang, X.; Wan, K.; Zhang, X.; Liu, X.; Wei, G., Peptide-engineered fluorescent nanomaterials: Structure design, function tailoring, and biomedical applications. *Small* **2021**, 17 (5), 2005578.
103. Kimmerlin, T.; Seebach, D., '100 years of peptide synthesis': Ligation methods for peptide and protein synthesis with applications to β-peptide assemblies. *The Journal of Peptide Research* **2005**, 65 (2), 229–260.

104. Agouridas, V.; El Mahdi, O.; Diemer, V.; Cargoët, M.; Monbaliu, J.-C. M.; Melnyk, O., Native chemical ligation and extended methods: Mechanisms, catalysis, scope, and limitations. *Chemical Reviews* **2019**, 119 (12), 7328–7443.
105. Thompson, R. E.; Chan, B.; Radom, L.; Jolliffe, K. A.; Payne, R. J., Chemoselective peptide ligation–desulfurization at aspartate. *Angewandte Chemie* **2013**, *125* (37), 9905–9909.
106. Roberts, K. E.; Cushing, P. R.; Boisguerin, P.; Madden, D. R.; Donald, B. R., Computational design of a PDZ domain peptide inhibitor that rescues CFTR activity. *PLoS Computational Biology* **2012**, *8* (4), e1002477.
107. Fremaux, J.; Venin, C.; Mauran, L.; Zimmer, R. H.; Guichard, G.; Goudreau, S. R., Peptide-oligourea hybrids analogue of GLP-1 with improved action in vivo. *Nature Communications* **2019**, 10 (1), 924.
108. Hawker, C. J.; Wooley, K. L., The convergence of synthetic organic and polymer chemistries. *Science* **2005**, 309 (5738), 1200–1205.
109. Vandermeulen, G. W.; Klok, H. A., Peptide/protein hybrid materials: Enhanced control of structure and improved performance through conjugation of biological and synthetic polymers. *Macromolecular Bioscience* **2004**, *4* (4), 383–398.
110. Čemažar, M.; Craik, D. J., Microwave-assisted Boc-solid phase peptide synthesis of cyclic cysteine-rich peptides. *Journal of Peptide Science: An Official Publication of the European Peptide Society* **2008**, 14 (6), 683–689.
111. Mándity, I. M.; Ötvös, S. B.; Szőlősi, G.; Fülöp, F., Harnessing the versatility of continuous-flow processes: Selective and efficient reactions. *The Chemical Record* **2016**, 16 (3), 1018–1033.
112. Yu, B.; Zhao, X.; Lee, L. J.; Lee, R. J., Targeted delivery systems for oligonucleotide therapeutics. *The AAPS Journal* **2009**, 11, 195–203.
113. Chen, L.; Hong, W.; Ren, W.; Xu, T.; Qian, Z.; He, Z., Recent progress in targeted delivery vectors based on biomimetic nanoparticles. *Signal Transduction and Targeted Therapy* **2021**, *6* (1), 225.
114. Wang, Y.; Li, S.; Wang, X.; Chen, Q.; He, Z.; Luo, C.; Sun, J., Smart transformable nanomedicines for cancer therapy. *Biomaterials* **2021**, *271*, 120737.
115. Newberry, R. W.; VanVeller, B.; Raines, R. T., Thioamides in the collagen triple helix. *Chemical Communications* **2015**, 51 (47), 9624–9627.
116. Huie, C. W.; Di, X., Chromatographic and electrophoretic methods for Lingzhi pharmacologically active components. *Journal of Chromatography B* **2004**, 812 (1–2), 241–257.
117. Devadasu, V. R., Evaluation of antioxidants encapsulated nanoparticles in animal models. University of Strathclyde, Strathclyde Institute of Pharmacy and Biomedical Sciences, 2011.
118. Zhu, B.-Y.; Mant, C. T.; Hodges, R. S., Hydrophilic-interaction chromatography of peptides on hydrophilic and strong cation-exchange columns. *Journal of Chromatography A* 1991, 548, 13–24.
119. Madadlou, A.; O'Sullivan, S.; Sheehan, D., Fast protein liquid chromatography. *Protein Chromatography: Methods and Protocols* 2011, 681, 439–447.
120. Malmström, J.; Lee, H.; Nesvizhskii, A. I.; Shteynberg, D.; Mohanty, S.; Brunner, E.; Ye, M.; Weber, G.; Eckerskorn, C.; Aebersold, R., Optimized peptide separation and identification for mass spectrometry based proteomics via free-flow electrophoresis. *Journal of Proteome Research* **2006**, 5 (9), 2241–2249.
121. Muttenthaler, M.; King, G. F.; Adams, D. J.; Alewood, P. F., Trends in peptide drug discovery. *Nature Reviews Drug Discovery* **2021**, 20 (4), 309–325.
122. Agarwal, P.; Goyal, A., A review on analyzers for mass spectrometry. *International Journal of Pharma and Bio Sciences* **2017**, 8 (4), 139–151.

123. Parasuraman, S.; Anish, R.; Balamurugan, S.; Muralidharan, S.; Kumar, K. J.; Vijayan, V., An overview of liquid chromatography-mass spectroscopy instrumentation. *Pharmaceutical Methods* 2014, 5 (2), 47–55.
124. Finehout, E. J.; Lee, K. H., An introduction to mass spectrometry applications in biological research. *Biochemistry and Molecular Biology Education* **2004**, 32 (2), 93–100.
125. Taulelle, F., NMR crystallography: Crystallochemical formula and space group selection. *Solid State Sciences* **2004**, 6 (10), 1053–1057.
126. Lankhorst, P. P.; Erkelens, C.; Haasnoot, C. A.; Altona, C., Carbon-13 NMR in conformational analysis of nudeic add fragments. Heteronuclear chemical shift correlation spectroscopy of RNA constitutents. *Nucleic Acids Research* **1983**, 11 (20), 7215–7230.
127. Dias, D. A.; Urban, S.; Roessner, U., A historical overview of natural products in drug discovery. *Metabolites* **2012**, 2 (2), 303–336.

3 Peptide-based nanostructures

3.1 INTRODUCTION TO PEPTIDE-BASED NANOSTRUCTURES

Elegant cell designs are the result of the convenience with which simple molecules can be used to construct complex structures. Peptide-based nanostructures are examples of forming supramolecular structures through the self-assembly of peptides.[1] To sustain cellular homeostasis and functioning, nature depends on the formation of supramolecular assembly of nucleic acids, proteins, and lipids. Through noncovalent interactions, such as hydrogen bonds, hydrophobic bonds, electrostatic interactions, van der Waals forces, and π-π stacking, molecules spontaneously organize into a specific structure known as a supramolecular assembly.[2] The resulting structures have numerous applications, including medication delivery, tissue engineering, and biosensors.[1] These properties concists of high degree of specificity and can be designed to have specific properties such as charge, hydrophobicity, and shape allowing peptides to self-assemble into a variety range of structures, as the following nanoribbons,[3] nanofibers,[4] and nanotubes.[5]

The peptide sequence determines the specific interactions that occur during self-assembly, which ultimately regulates the final structure. Peptides with complementary sequences interact to form β-sheets, which can then stack to form nanofibers or nanotubes. Peptides with amphiphilic properties can form micelles or nanoparticles (NPs).[6]

Peptide-based nanostructures have several advantages over traditional nanostructures, including biocompatibility, biodegradability, and the ability to target specific cells or tissues.[7] Peptides are designed to have specific targeting sequences that allow them to bind to specific cells or tissues. This can be useful for drug delivery, as it allows drugs to be delivered directly to the site of action, reducing side effects and increasing efficacy.[8]

Peptide-based nanostructures can also be used for tissue engineering. By mimicking the extracellular matrix (ECM), peptide-based nanofibers can provide a scaffold for cells to grow and differentiate. The nanofibers can also be functionalized with specific peptides or growth factors to promote cell growth and differentiation.[9]

In addition to drug delivery and tissue engineering, peptide-based nanostructures have several other applications. They can be used as biosensors to detect specific molecules or pathogens.[10] Peptide-based NPs can also be used for imaging, as they can be functionalized with contrast agents that allow them to be

Peptide-based nanostructures

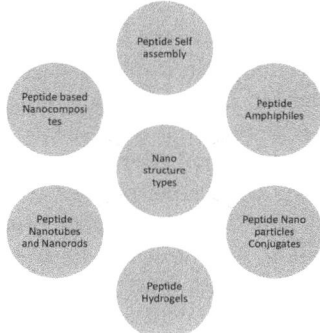

FIGURE 3.1 Classification of peptide-based nanostructures.

visualized using imaging techniques such as magnetic resonance imaging (MRI) or computed tomography (CT).[11]

Peptide-based nanostructures are a relatively recent field, and there can be much research to be done to fully understand the properties and potential applications of these structures. However, the potential benefits of these structures are significant, and they are likely to in the future; nanotechnology will play an increasingly essential role in medicine and other sectors.

Hereby, peptide-based nanostructures have emerged as an intriguing foundation for a variety of applications. Their ability to self-assemble into a wide range of structures and their biocompatibility, biodegradability, and ability to target specific cells or tissues make them an attractive alternative to traditional nanostructures. Peptide-based nanostructures have the ability to revolutionize drug delivery, tissue engineering, biosensors, and imaging, and further research in this field is likely to uncover new and exciting applications, with various types as shown in Figure 3.1 of nanostructures incorporated peptide.

3.2 PEPTIDE SELF-ASSEMBLY

Self-assembly refers to the process through which peptides spontaneously organize into structures, such as nanofibers, nanotubes, or NPs. Because of their ability to generate noncovalent interactions such as hydrogen bonds, electrostatic interactions, hydrophobic interactions, π-π stacking, and van der Waals forces, building blocks are adaptable for self-assembly. These interactions can occur between peptide backbones, side chains, or both, based on the peptide's particular arrangement sequence. The resulting supramolecular structures have unique physical and chemical properties that depend on the length, sequence, and concentration of the peptides.[2]

Peptide self-assembly is a bottom-up approach to building nanostructures.[12] Unlike top-down approaches, which involve carving or etching materials to create nanostructures, self-assembly is a more efficient and scalable approach. The self-assembly process is also highly selective and controllable, allowing the production of complex structures with specific sizes, shapes, and functions.[13]

The self-assembly of peptides can occur through several different mechanisms. One common mechanism is the formation of β-sheets,[14] which are planar structures that form when peptide chains fold back on themselves and hydrogen bonds form between adjacent chains. β-Sheets can stack up to create nanofibers or nanotubes, with the peptide side chains exposed on the structure's surface.[15]

Another mechanism of peptide self-assembly is through the formation of α-helices. α-Helices are helical structures that form when a peptide chain coils around itself, with hydrogen bonds forming between the amino and carboxy termini of the chain. They can associate with each other to form coiled coils, which can further self-assemble into higher-order structures.[16]

Peptide self-assembly has several advantages over other methods of building nanostructures. Peptides are biocompatible, biodegradable, and nontoxic, making them ideal for use in biomedical applications. Peptides can also be designed with specific properties, such as charge, hydrophobicity, and shape, to control their self-assembly into specific structures. This enables the development of structures with specific purposes, such as drug delivery, tissue engineering, or biosensors.

While a peptide self-assembly is a potent tool for the production of nanostructures with specific properties and functions, the unique physical and chemical properties of peptides allow for the precise control of self-assembly; consequently, they are suitable for a broad range of applications. Peptide self-assembly has the potential to revolutionize fields such as drug delivery, tissue engineering, and biosensors, and further research in this area is likely to uncover new and exciting applications.[9]

3.3 PEPTIDE AMPHIPHILIC

Peptide amphiphiles (PAs) are a class of molecules that combine both peptide and amphiphilic properties. They typically consist of a hydrophobic tail, a spacer region, and a hydrophilic head (an alkyl chain, lipid, polymer, or polypeptide), which contains a peptide sequence.[17] The hydrophobic tail is usually composed of a fatty acid or a lipid, while the hydrophilic head can vary depending on the desired application.[18]

Pas' amphiphilic nature allows them to self-assemble into a wide range of nanostructures such as micelles, nanofibers, and NPs. The self-assembly is the hydrophobic effect that causes the hydrophobic tails to collect together inside the structure, leaving the hydrophilic heads exposed on the surface.

The peptide sequence in PAs can be designed to have specific properties, such as charge, hydrophobicity, and shape, which can control the self-assembly of the molecule.[19] The peptide sequence can also be designed to mimic specific biological molecules, such as growth factors or ECM proteins, to promote specific biological functions.[20]

PAs have numerous potential biomedical applications, including medication delivery, tissue engineering, and regenerative medicine. In drug delivery, PAs are designed to encapsulate drugs and deliver them to precise cells or tissues. The hydrophilic head of the PA can be imbued with targeted molecules, such as antibodies or peptides, to increase the specificity of drug delivery. The hydrophobic tail can also be designed to release the drug in a controlled manner, prolonging its therapeutic effect.[8]

In fields such as tissue engineering and regenerative medicine, PAs are applied to create scaffolds for cell growth and differentiation. The hydrophilic head of the PA is functionalized with specific peptides or growth factors to promote cell adhesion, proliferation, and differentiation. The self-assembly of PAs into nanofibers or NPs can also provide a structure for cells to attach to and organize around.

PAs can also be used as biosensors, as the self-assembled nanostructures can be functionalized with specific peptides or antibodies to detect specific molecules or pathogens. The sensitivity and specificity of the biosensor can be increased by modifying the peptide sequence to bind with high affinity to the target molecule.[21]

Thus, we understand that PAs are a versatile class of molecules with a wide range of potential applications in biomedicine. The combination of peptide and amphiphilic properties allows for the precise control of self-assembly and the ability to mimic specific biological molecules. PAs have the potential to revolutionize drug delivery, tissue engineering, and biosensing, and further research in this area is likely to uncover new and exciting applications.[22]

3.4 PEPTIDE-BASED NPS

Peptide-based NPs are a type of nanoscale materials that are made up of peptides.[23] They have unique physical, chemical, and biological properties that make them promising for various biomedical applications, including imaging, sensing carrier-mediated drug delivery, tissue engineering, antimicrobial agents, imaging tools, energy storage, biomineralization, and membrane protein stabilization.[24]

Peptide-based NPs can be designed by modifying the sequence of the peptide to control their size, shape, surface charge, and stability. They can be synthesized through various techniques, such as self-assembly, coacervation, or layer-by-layer assembly.[25] Once synthesized, these NPs can be further functionalized with various moieties, such as targeting ligands, imaging agents, or therapeutic drugs (Figure 3.2).

One of the most important benefits of peptide-based NPs is their biocompatibility and biodegradability. Peptides are naturally occurring molecules found in living organisms, and therefore, they are considered to be safe for biomedical applications. The biodegradability of these NPs makes them appealing for drug delivery applications, as they can be easily metabolized and cleared from the body without causing any harm. One such example is our study involving XLAsp-P2 conjugated with cellulose acetate for wound healing applications. This formulation demonstrated effective inhibition against four pathogenic microorganisms: *Escherichia coli* (ATCC 25922), *Pseudomonas aeruginosa* (ATCC 27853), *Staphylococcus aureus* (ATCC 25923), and *Bacillus cereus* (ATCC 11778).[26]

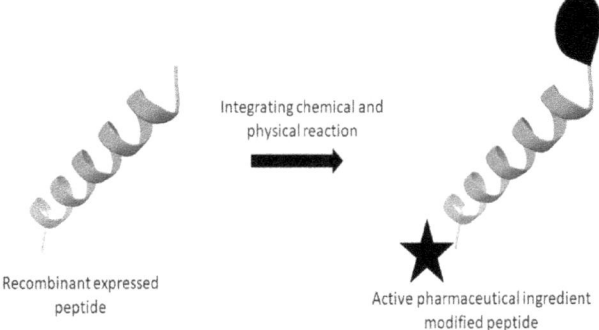

FIGURE 3.2 Late-stage peptide modification that is selective and efficient required for the creation of contemporary peptide-based medicines.

To increase selectivity, NPs can be functionalized with targeted ligands such as antibodies, peptides, or aptamers and selectivity towards specific cells or tissues.[27] This allows for the delivery of therapeutic drugs directly to the site of action, reducing the risk of off-target effects and improving the efficacy of the treatment.[28]

In addition to drug delivery, peptide-based NPs can also be used for imaging and sensing applications. They can be functionalized with various imaging agents, such as fluorescent dyes or magnetic NPs, to enable noninvasive visualization of cells or tissues.[29] Peptide-based NPs can also be used as biosensors, as they can be functionalized with specific peptides or antibodies to detect specific molecules or pathogens.

Overall, peptide-based NPs are a promising class of materials with a wide range of potential applications in biomedicine. Their biocompatibility, biodegradability, and ability to be functionalized make them appealing for medication administration, imaging, and sensing applications. As research in this field continues, new and innovative applications for peptide-based NPs will likely be discovered.

3.5 PEPTIDE-BASED HYDROGELS

Peptide-based hydrogels are a type of hydrogel made up of peptides that can self-assemble to form a three-dimensional (3D) network structure capable of retaining large amounts of water. Hydrogels are important materials in biomedical applications because of their ability to resemble ECM, providing a supportive environment for cells and tissues.[30]

Peptide-based hydrogels can be designed by modifying the sequence of the peptide to control their physical and mechanical properties, as well as their biocompatibility and bioactivity. They can be synthesized using various techniques, such as self-assembly, covalent cross-linking, or physical cross-linking.

One of the significant advantages of peptide-based hydrogels is their biocompatibility and ability to mimic the ECM. Peptide-based hydrogels can be designed to have similar properties to the ECM, providing a supportive environment for cell growth and tissue regeneration.[31] Additionally, peptide-based hydrogels can be functionalized with various biomolecules, such as growth factors or signaling peptides, to promote cell adhesion, proliferation, and differentiation.[32]

Peptide-based hydrogels can also be used for drug delivery applications, which can be designed to encapsulate therapeutic drugs and release them in a controlled manner. The peptide sequence can be modified to control the release rate, allowing for the sustained release of drugs over an extended period, improving the efficacy of the treatment.[33]

Peptide-based hydrogels can also be used for tissue engineering applications. They can be designed to create scaffolds for cell growth and differentiation, mimicking the native tissue environment. Peptide-based hydrogels can be functionalized with specific peptides or growth factors to promote cell adhesion, proliferation, and differentiation.[34]

In addition to drug delivery and tissue engineering, peptide-based hydrogels can also be used for sensing and diagnostic applications. They can be functionalized with specific peptides or antibodies to detect specific molecules or pathogens, making them useful for biosensing applications.[35]

Peptide-based hydrogels are a promising class of materials with a wide range of potential applications in biomedicine. Their biocompatibility, ability to mimic the ECM, and ability to be functionalized make them appealing for medication delivery and tissue engineering, and sensing applications.

3.6 PEPTIDE NANOTUBES AND NANORODS

Peptide nanotubes and nanorods are a type of nanoscale materials made up of peptides that self-assemble into long, thin structures. Carbon nanotubes (CNTs) are cylinder-shaped macromolecules that can grow up to 20 cm in length and possess a radius as small as a few nanometers.[36] The geometric arrangement of the carbon atoms at the cylinder seam essentially gives rise to the classification of nanotubes as armchairs ($n=m$) or zigzag ($m=0$). Nanotubes with mn are chiral, even though both of these forms of tubes have mirror symmetry. Both right-handed and left-handed enantiomers of the latter class of tubes are present.[37] The chiral vector of a nanotube, which is represented by the chiral indices (n, m), can be used to entirely specify the structure of a nanotube dependent on the tube axis's direction concerning the hexagonal lattice.[38]

3.6.1 Preparation of nanotubes

Bundles formed up of up to hundreds of solitary nanotubes are constantly the product of large-scale nanotube manufacturing processes. However, it is better to have independently scattered nanotubes rather than bundles to allow simple access to chemical reagents.[39] The individual tubes are then enclosed with a

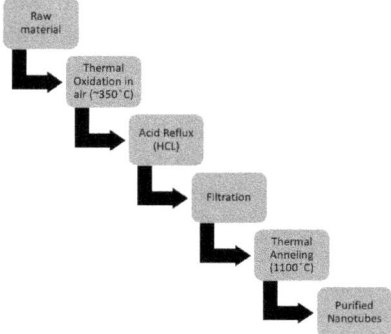

FIGURE 3.3 The purification process for single-walled CNTs.

detergent shell after the CNTs are subjected to an effective ultrasonic treatment for this purpose in an aqueous surfactant solution. It is important to emphasize that the experimental setup must be properly managed because intense ultrasonication can seriously harm the tube walls[36,39]; hence, purification steps (Figure 3.3) are required.

These structures are unique and have physical and chemical features that make them appealing for an assortment of biomedical applications, including drug delivery, imaging, and tissue engineering.

Peptide nanotubes and nanorods can be designed by modifying the sequence of the peptide to control their size, shape, surface charge, and stability. They can be synthesized through various techniques, such as self-assembly or template-assisted synthesis.[40] One of the most significant advantages of peptide nanotubes and nanorods is their high aspect ratio (Figure 3.4). These structures are long and thin, allowing them to penetrate deep into tissues and cells, making them attractive for drug delivery applications. Additionally, their high aspect ratio provides a significant amount of surface area for functionalization, enabling the attachment of various biomolecules for targeting or sensing applications.[41]

Peptide nanotubes and nanorods can also be used for imaging and sensing applications. They can be functionalized with various imaging agents, such as fluorescent dyes or magnetic NPs, to enable noninvasive visualization of cells or tissues. Peptide nanotubes and nanorods can also be used as biosensors, as they can be functionalized with specific peptides or antibodies to detect specific molecules or pathogens.[41]

In addition to drug delivery and imaging, peptide nanotubes and nanorods can also be used for tissue engineering applications. They can be designed to create scaffolds for cell growth and differentiation, mimicking the native tissue environment. Peptide nanotubes and nanorods can be functionalized with specific peptides or growth factors to promote cell adhesion, proliferation, and differentiation.

While nanotubes and nanorods are a promising class of materials with a wide range of potential applications in biomedicine. Their beneficial aspect ratio, biocompatibility, and functionalization ability make them attractive to various

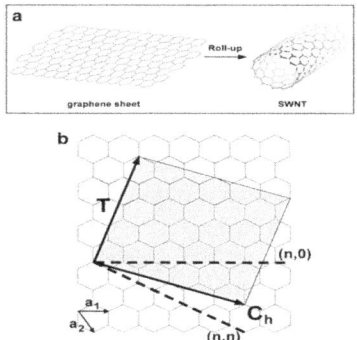

FIGURE 3.4 Rollup of a graphene sheet leading to the three different types of CNT. Reprinted with permission from ref.[42] Copyright © 2000 American Chemical Society.

applications. Materials can transport insoluble pharmaceuticals because of their higher water solubility, which eliminates the requirement for hazardous organic solvents and associated negative side effects. The release kinetics of nanocarriers can be tailored utilizing external stimuli like heat and ultrasound as well as environmental factors like pH.[28] This benefit of controlled release minimizes drug buildup in other healthy tissues and organs, reducing drug-related systemic toxicity by preventing premature dissociation of the drug from the nanoshell before it reaches the tumor site.

3.6.2 Difference between peptide nanotubes and nanorods

Peptide nanotubes and nanorods are two different types of nanoscale materials made up of peptides that self-assemble into long, thin structures. While they share some similarities, such as their high aspect ratio and potential biomedical applications, they differ in their shape and size.[43]

Peptide nanotubes are long, cylindrical structures with a diameter ranging from a few nanometers to several micrometers and a length that can reach up to several hundred micrometers.[44] They are typically formed by the self-assembly of peptide molecules, and their internal diameter can be controlled by changing the peptide sequence or the conditions of the self-assembly process. Peptide nanotubes can have a variety of surface functional groups, which can be used to attach other molecules or NPs for targeted drug delivery or sensing applications.[45]

Nanotubes, on the other hand, do not have perfect architectures; instead, they have synthesis-related flaws. An average defect site contains 1–3% of the carbon atoms in a nanotube.[46] The so-called Stone-Wales defect, also known as a 7-5-5-7 defect because it consists of two pairs of five-membered and seven-membered rings, is a type of defect that is frequently found. The local deformation of the graphitic sidewall caused by a Stone-Wales defect increases the curvature in this area. The connection within two five-membered rings has the strongest curvature, which favors addition reactions at the carbon-carbon double bonds in these locations.[47]

In contrast, peptide nanorods are elongated structures with a diameter ranging from several nanometers to a few hundred nanometers and a length that can reach up to several micrometers. They are typically generated as a result of the self-assembly of peptide molecules into a rodlike structure (Figure 3.5). The shape and size of peptide nanorods can be controlled by changing the peptide sequence or the conditions of the self-assembly process.[48] Peptide nanorods also have a variety of surface functional groups, which can be used to attach other molecules or NPs for targeted drug delivery or sensing applications.[49]

Gold nanorods (GNRs), which have special shape-dependent optical properties, have sparked attention across the globe in the field of biomedicine (Figure 3.7). Two separate plasmon bands can be seen in these nanorods.[48] The first is a transverse plasmon band in the visible spectrum, , and the second is a longitudinal plasmon band in the near-infrared (IR) spectrum. These particular properties show promise for the development of novel optically active chemicals that carry out both photothermal cancer treatment and light-mediated imaging.[50]

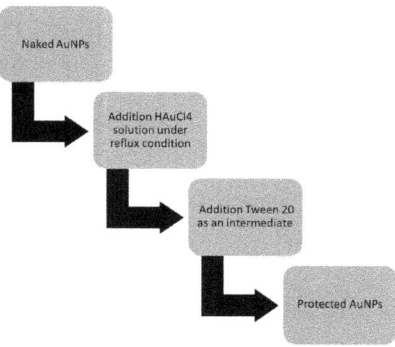

FIGURE 3.5 Flowchart of two-phase synthesis of AuNPs.

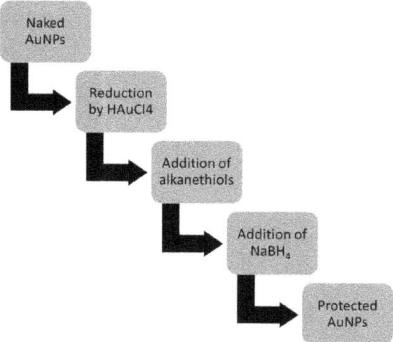

FIGURE 3.6 Flowchart of citrate-stabilized AuNPs.

Turkevich and colleagues proposed a synthetic method for producing gold NPs (AuNPs) in 1951 by exposing hydrogen tetrachloroaurate (HAuCl$_4$) to citric acid in boiling water.[51] Citrate functions as both a reducing and a stabilizing agent in this process, as shown in Figure 3.6. Later, Frens improved on this approach by altering the gold-to-citrate ratio, which allowed for exact control of particle size. This well-established method has been widely used to prepare aqueous solutions containing moderately stable spherical AuNPs with sizes ranging from 10 to 20 nm. Nonetheless, it's worth mentioning that this approach can also be used to create larger AuNPs, such as those with diameters of 100 nm. A substantial problem occurs during the functionalization of these citrate-stabilized AuNPs with thiolate ligands in the form of irreversible aggregation. Various techniques have been suggested to overcome this issue. As shown in Figure 3.6, one strategy involves using a surfactant, namely Tween 20, before the modification phase to successfully prevent aggregation. A two-step functionalization approach using thioctic acid as an intermediate has also been proposed. However, due to the demand for significant dilution in these tactics, establishing large-scale manufacturing might be difficult.[52]

Brust and Schriffin achieved a breakthrough in AuNP synthesis in 1994 when they used a biphasic reduction process with tetraoctylammonium bromide (TOAB) as the phase transfer reagent and sodium borohydride (NaBH$_4$) as the reducing agent to create organic soluble alkanethiol-stabilized AuNPs (Figure 3.7).[15,53] By changing reaction variables such as gold-to-thiol ratio, reduction rate, and reaction temperature, this approach yields low dispersity AuNPs ranging from 1.5 to 5 nm.[16] Because of the synergistic effect of the strong thiol-gold contacts and van der Waals attractions between the surrounding ligands, these alkanethiol-protected AuNPs are more stable than most other AuNPs. These NPs are good precursors for subsequent functionalization since they may be fully dried and redispersed in solution without aggregation.[54]

While both peptide nanotubes and nanorods share some similarities, they differ in their shape and size, which can impact their properties and potential applications. Peptide nanotubes are generally larger than peptide nanorods and have a larger internal diameter, which may make them ideal for a variety of applications

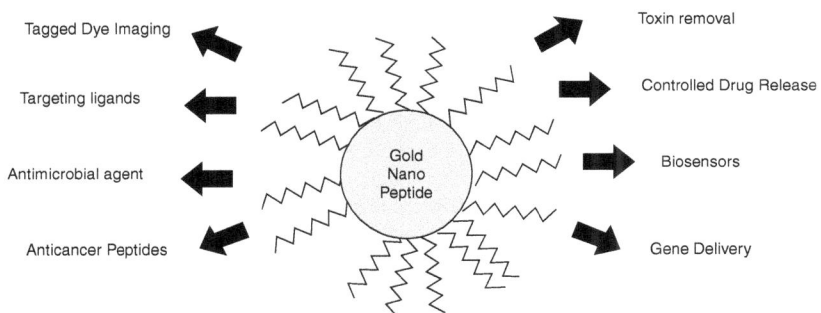

FIGURE 3.7 Gold-embedded nanoparticle applications.

including tissue engineering. Peptide nanorods, on the other hand, have a smaller diameter, which may make them more suitable for applications such as drug delivery, where they can penetrate cells more easily. Ultimately, the choice of whether to use peptide nanotubes or nanorods will depend on the specific application and desired properties.

3.7 PEPTIDE-BASED NANOCOMPOSITES

Peptide-based nanocomposites are a type of material that combines peptides with other nanomaterials to create hybrid structures with unique properties.[55] Peptide-based nanocomposites can be formed through various techniques, such as self-assembly, covalent bonding, or physical mixing. The choice of technique depends on the properties desired for the resulting nanocomposite. For example, self-assembly can be used to create nanocomposites with precise control over the size and morphology of the structure. Covalent bonding can be used to create stable, long-lasting nanocomposites, while physical mixing can be used to create easily synthesized and scalable nanocomposites.[56]

The incorporation of other nanomaterials into peptide-based nanocomposites can enhance their properties and functionality. For example, the incorporation of magnetic NPs into a peptide-based nanocomposite can create a magnetic nanocomposite that can be guided by an external magnetic field for targeted drug delivery.[57] Similarly, the incorporation of AuNPs into a peptide-based nanocomposite can create a plasmonic nanocomposite with distinct optical characteristics that can be employed in sensing applications.[58]

Peptide-based nanocomposites can also be used for tissue engineering applications. By incorporating peptides that mimic the ECM of a specific tissue, peptide-based nanocomposites can provide a suitable scaffold for cell growth and differentiation. In addition, the incorporation of other nanomaterials, such as hydroxyapatite or calcium phosphate, can enhance the mechanical properties of the nanocomposite, making it more suitable for load-bearing applications.[59]

Peptide-based nanocomposites are a promising class of materials with a wide range of potential applications in biomedicine. Their ability to be functionalized with other nanomaterials can enhance their properties and functionality, making NPs appealing for applications like medication delivery, tissue engineering, and sensing.

3.8 CHARACTERIZATION OF PEPTIDE-BASED NANOSTRUCTURES

Characterization is critical to develop peptide-based nanostructures for understanding their properties and potential applications. There are several techniques available to characterize peptide-based nanostructures, including microscopy, spectroscopy, and rheology.

Microscopy techniques, such as transmission electron microscopy (TEM) and scanning electron microscopy (SEM), can be used to visualize the morphology, size, and surface characteristics of peptide-based nanostructures. TEM can provide high-resolution images of the nanomaterial's interior structure, while SEM is capable of providing surface topography and morphology data. Atomic force microscopy (AFM) can also be used to image the surface of the nanomaterial and provide information about its mechanical properties.[60]

Spectroscopic techniques, such as IR spectroscopy, Raman spectroscopy, and circular dichroism (CD), can be used to characterize the chemical composition and structure of peptide-based nanostructures. IR spectroscopy can provide information about the functional groups present in the nanomaterial, while Raman spectroscopy may reveal information related to the nanomaterial's vibrations at the molecular level.[61] CD spectroscopy can be used to determine the secondary structure of the peptide in the nanomaterial.[62]

Rheological techniques, such as oscillatory rheometry and shear rheometry, may be used to quantify the mechanical qualities of peptide-based hydrogels. These techniques can provide information about the elasticity, viscosity, and shear modulus of the hydrogel, which are critical for activities including tissue engineering.[63]

Other techniques, such as X-ray diffraction (XRD), small-angle X-ray scattering (SAXS), and dynamic light scattering (DLS). It is additionally feasible to study the structure and characteristics of peptide-based nanostructures.[64] XRD can provide information about the crystal structure of the nanomaterial, while SAXS could be used to calculate the size and shape of the nanomaterial. The size distribution of a nanomaterial in solution can be measured using DLS.[65]

Overall, a combination of these techniques can provide a comprehensive characterization of peptide-based nanostructures, which is essential for understanding their properties and potential applications. The technique used is determined by the qualities of the nanomaterial that need to be characterized, and multiple techniques may need to be used to obtain a complete understanding of the nanomaterial.

3.9 APPLICATIONS OF PEPTIDE-BASED NANOSTRUCTURES

Peptide-based nanostructures have numerous prospective uses in various fields, including biomedicine, nanotechnology, and materials science. Among the most potential applications of peptide-based nanostructures include:

1. Drug delivery: Peptide-based NPs can be employed as medication carriers for attacking specific cells or tissues in the body, increasing the effectiveness of the drug as well as minimizing adverse effects. These NPs may be modified with targeted ligands like antibodies or peptides to selectively bind to specific cell receptors.[66]
2. Tissue engineering: Peptide-based hydrogels can be used as supports to aid in growth and regeneration of tissues. These hydrogels could be designed to impersonate the ECM of specific tissues, providing an appropriate setting for cell growth and differentiation.

3. Imaging: MRI, CT, and fluorescence imaging can all benefit from the use of peptide-based NPs as contrast agents. To improve their imaging properties, these NPs can be functionalized with imaging agents such as fluorescent dyes or magnetic NPs.
4. Sensing: Peptide-based nanostructures can be used as biosensors to detect specific molecules or biomarkers. These nanostructures can be functionalized with recognition elements, such as peptides or antibodies, to selectively bind to the target molecule and produce a signal.
5. Energy conversion and storage: Peptide-based nanostructures can be used in energy conversion and storage devices, such as solar cells and batteries. These nanostructures can be functionalized with materials such as graphene or CNTs to enhance their electrical conductivity and energy storage properties.
6. Environmental applications: Peptide-based nanostructures can be used for environmental applications, such as water purification and pollution control. These nanostructures can be functionalized with materials such as NPs or enzymes to enhance their pollutant removal properties.

In summary, peptide-based nanostructures have numerous potential uses in a variety of sectors. Their distinguishing characteristics, including biocompatibility, self-assembly, and functionalization, make them appealing for a wide range of applications, including drug administration and tissue engineering, imaging, sensing, energy conversion and storage, and environmental applications. It is expected that as study in this sector continues, new and innovative applications for peptide-based nanostructures will be discovered.

3.10 FUTURE PROSPECTS OF PEPTIDE-BASED NANOSTRUCTURES

Peptide-based nanostructures have shown great potential in various applications, and ongoing research is expected to lead to even more exciting developments and applications in the future. Here are some of the potential future prospects of peptide-based nanostructures:

1. Precision medicine: Peptide-based nanostructures have the potential to revolutionize precision medicine, which is a branch of medicine in which therapies are personalized to individual patients depending on their specific genetic and molecular characteristics. Peptide-based nanostructures can be functionalized with targeting ligands to selectively deliver drugs to specific cells or tissues, and their properties can be customized to match the needs of individual patients.[67]
2. 3D printing: Peptide-based hydrogels could be utilized for 3D printing of complex tissues and organs. This could lead to the creation of patient-specific organs and tissues for transplantation, reducing the need for donor organs and minimizing the risk of rejection.[68]

3. **Wearable technology:** Peptide-based nanostructures could be incorporated into wearable devices, such as smart clothing or sensors, to monitor health status and deliver personalized treatments. This could have applications in healthcare, sports, and military settings.[69]
4. **Nanoelectronics:** Peptide-based nanostructures can be utilized to construct nanoelectronics, such as nanoscale transistors and sensors. These structures could potentially enable the development of faster and more efficient computing devices.[70]
5. **Environmental remediation:** Peptide-based nanostructures can be used for environmental remediation, such as removing pollutants from soil and water. Functionalized peptide-based nanostructures could target specific pollutants, enhancing the effectiveness of remediation efforts.[71]
6. **Biocatalysis:** Peptide-based nanostructures could be used as biocatalysts for various industrial processes. These structures could potentially replace conventional catalysts, which can be expensive and environmentally harmful such as the enzymatic activity of peptide fibrils as well as the catalytic abilities of supramolecular gels, including those of peptide-based molecules in organocatalysis.[72]

In conclusion, peptide-based nanostructures have a promising future with many potential applications in various fields. Ongoing research will likely lead to new and exciting developments, further expanding the possibilities for the use of peptide-based nanostructures in various fields.

3.11 PRACTICAL QUESTIONS

1. How do peptide-based nanostructures self-assemble, and what are the key driving forces behind their formation?
2. What are the various methods for fabricating and manipulating peptide-based nanostructures?
3. Explain the different types of peptide-based nanostructures, including nanotubes, nanofibers, NPs, and peptide-based hydrogels.
4. How can researchers modify the surface chemistry of these nanostructures to improve biocompatibility and targeting capabilities?
5. What are the challenges and prospects in the field of peptide-based nanostructures?

REFERENCES

1. Kim, J.; Narayana, A.; Patel, S.; Sahay, G., Advances in intracellular delivery through supramolecular self-assembly of oligonucleotides and peptides. *Theranostics* 2019, 9 (11), 3191.
2. Caulder, D. L.; Raymond, K. N., Supermolecules by design. *Accounts of Chemical Research* 1999, 32 (11), 975–982.
3. Wang, M.; Wang, J.; Zhou, P.; Deng, J.; Zhao, Y.; Sun, Y.; Yang, W.; Wang, D.; Li, Z.; Hu, X., Nanoribbons self-assembled from short peptides demonstrate the formation of polar zippers between β-sheets. *Nature Communications* 2018, 9 (1), 5118.

4. Hartgerink, J. D.; Beniash, E.; Stupp, S. I., Self-assembly and mineralization of peptide-amphiphile nanofibers. *Science* 2001, *294* (5547), 1684–1688.
5. Brendel, J. C.; Sanchis, J.; Catrouillet, S.; Czuba, E.; Chen, M. Z.; Long, B. M.; Nowell, C.; Johnston, A.; Jolliffe, K. A.; Perrier, S., Secondary self-assembly of supramolecular nanotubes into tubisomes and their activity on cells. *Angewandte Chemie International Edition* 2018, *57* (51), 16678–16682.
6. Hu, X.; Liao, M.; Gong, H.; Zhang, L.; Cox, H.; Waigh, T. A.; Lu, J. R., Recent advances in short peptide self-assembly: From rational design to novel applications. *Current Opinion in Colloid & Interface Science* 2020, *45*, 1–13.
7. Bhatia, T.; Gupta, G. D.; Kurmi, B. D.; Singh, D., Role of solid lipid nanoparticles for the delivery of Lipophilic drugs and herbal medicines in the treatment of pulmonary hypertension. *Pharmaceutical Nanotechnology* 2022, *10* (5), 342–353.
8. Zhang, Z.; Ai, S.; Yang, Z.; Li, X., Peptide-based supramolecular hydrogels for local drug delivery. *Advanced Drug Delivery Reviews* 2021, *174*, 482–503.
9. Wang, Y. L.; Lin, S. P.; Nelli, S. R.; Zhan, F. K.; Cheng, H.; Lai, T. S.; Yeh, M. Y.; Lin, H. C.; Hung, S. C., Self-assembled peptide-based hydrogels as scaffolds for proliferation and multi-differentiation of mesenchymal stem cells. *Macromolecular Bioscience* 2017, *17* (4), 1600192.
10. Puiu, M.; Bala, C., Peptide-based biosensors: From self-assembled interfaces to molecular probes in electrochemical assays. *Bioelectrochemistry* 2018, *120*, 66–75.
11. Qi, G. B.; Gao, Y. J.; Wang, L.; Wang, H., Self-assembled peptide-based nanomaterials for biomedical imaging and therapy. *Advanced Materials* 2018, *30* (22), 1703444.
12. Gazit, E., Self-assembled peptide nanostructures: The design of molecular building blocks and their technological utilization. *Chemical Society Reviews* 2007, *36* (8), 1263–1269.
13. Seeman, N. C.; Belcher, A. M., Emulating biology: Building nanostructures from the bottom up. *Proceedings of the National Academy of Sciences* 2002, *99* (suppl_2), 6451–6455.
14. Zhao, Y.; Wang, J.; Deng, L.; Zhou, P.; Wang, S.; Wang, Y.; Xu, H.; Lu, J. R., Tuning the self-assembly of short peptides via sequence variations. *Langmuir* 2013, *29* (44), 13457–13464.
15. Rubinstein, I.; Eliash, R.; Bolbach, G.; Weissbuch, I.; Lahav, M., Racemic β sheets in biochirogenesis. *Angewandte Chemie International Edition* 2007, *46* (20), 3710–3713.
16. Woolfson, D. N., Building fibrous biomaterials from α-helical and collagen-like coiled-coil peptides. *Peptide Science: Original Research on Biomolecules* 2010, *94* (1), 118–127.
17. Versluis, F.; Marsden, H. R.; Kros, A., Power struggles in peptide-amphiphile nanostructures. *Chemical Society Reviews* 2010, *39* (9), 3434–3444.
18. M Leite, D.; Barbu, E.; J Pilkington, G.; Lalatsa, A., Peptide self-assemblies for drug delivery. *Current Topics in Medicinal Chemistry* 2015, *15* (22), 2277–2289.
19. Cui, H.; Webber, M. J.; Stupp, S. I., Self-assembly of peptide amphiphiles: From molecules to nanostructures to biomaterials. *Peptide Science: Original Research on Biomolecules* 2010, *94* (1), 1–18.
20. Fercana, G. R.; Yerneni, S.; Billaud, M.; Hill, J. C.; VanRyzin, P.; Richards, T. D.; Sicari, B. M.; Johnson, S. A.; Badylak, S. F.; Campbell, P. G., Perivascular extracellular matrix hydrogels mimic native matrix microarchitecture and promote angiogenesis via basic fibroblast growth factor. *Biomaterials* 2017, *123*, 142–154.

21. Feyzizarnagh, H.; Yoon, D. Y.; Goltz, M.; Kim, D. S., Peptide nanostructures in biomedical technology. *Wiley Interdisciplinary Reviews: Nanomedicine and Nanobiotechnology* 2016, 8 (5), 730–743.
22. Chang, H.; Li, C.; Huang, R.; Su, R.; Qi, W.; He, Z., Amphiphilic hydrogels for biomedical applications. *Journal of Materials Chemistry B* 2019, 7 (18), 2899–2910.
23. Tornesello, A. L.; Tagliamonte, M.; Tornesello, M. L.; Buonaguro, F. M.; Buonaguro, L., Nanoparticles to improve the efficacy of peptide-based cancer vaccines. *Cancers* 2020, *12* (4), 1049.
24. Zelzer, M.; Ulijn, R. V., Next-generation peptide nanomaterials: Molecular networks, interfaces and supramolecular functionality. *Chemical Society Reviews* 2010, 39 (9), 3351–3357.
25. Wang, J.; Liu, K.; Xing, R.; Yan, X., Peptide self-assembly: Thermodynamics and kinetics. *Chemical Society Reviews* 2016, 45 (20), 5589–5604.
26. Selvaraj, S.; Perera, M.; Yapa, P.; Munaweera, I.; Perera, I. C.; Senapathi, T.; Weerasinghe, L. In vitro analysis of XLAsp-P2 peptide loaded cellulose acetate nanofiber for wound healing. *Journal of Pharmaceutical Sciences* 2024.
27. Gu, F. X.; Karnik, R.; Wang, A. Z.; Alexis, F.; Levy-Nissenbaum, E.; Hong, S.; Langer, R. S.; Farokhzad, O. C., Targeted nanoparticles for cancer therapy. *Nano Today* 2007, 2 (3), 14–21.
28. Srinivasan, M.; Rajabi, M.; Mousa, S. A., Multifunctional nanomaterials and their applications in drug delivery and cancer therapy. *Nanomaterials* 2015, *5* (4), 1690–1703.
29. Veiga, N.; Diesendruck, Y.; Peer, D., Targeted nanomedicine: Lessons learned and future directions. *Journal of Controlled Release* 2023, 355, 446–457.
30. Henderson, T. M.; Ladewig, K.; Haylock, D. N.; McLean, K. M.; O'Connor, A. J., Cryogels for biomedical applications. *Journal of Materials Chemistry B* 2013, 1 (21), 2682–2695.
31. Hussey, G. S.; Dziki, J. L.; Badylak, S. F., Extracellular matrix-based materials for regenerative medicine. *Nature Reviews Materials* 2018, 3 (7), 159–173.
32. Zhu, J., Bioactive modification of poly (ethylene glycol) hydrogels for tissue engineering. *Biomaterials* 2010, *31* (17), 4639–4656.
33. Guan, T.; Li, J.; Chen, C.; Liu, Y., Self-assembling peptide-based hydrogels for wound tissue repair. *Advanced Science* 2022, *9* (10), 2104165.
34. Zhu, J.; Han, H.; Ye, T.-T.; Li, F.-X.; Wang, X.-L.; Yu, J.-Y.; Wu, D.-Q., Biodegradable and pH sensitive peptide based hydrogel as controlled release system for antibacterial wound dressing application. *Molecules* 2018, *23* (12), 3383.
35. Yadav, N.; Chauhan, M. K.; Chauhan, V. S., Short to ultrashort peptide-based hydrogels as a platform for biomedical applications. *Biomaterials Science* 2020, 8 (1), 84–100.
36. Balasubramanian, K.; Burghard, M., Chemically functionalized carbon nanotubes. *Small* 2005, *1* (2), 180–192.
37. Iijima, S.; Ichihashi, T., Single-shell carbon nanotubes of 1-nm diameter. *Nature* 1993, *363* (6430), 603–605.
38. O'connell, M. J.; Bachilo, S. M.; Huffman, C. B.; Moore, V. C.; Strano, M. S.; Haroz, E. H.; Rialon, K. L.; Boul, P. J.; Noon, W. H.; Kittrell, C., Band gap fluorescence from individual single-walled carbon nanotubes. *Science* 2002, *297* (5581), 593–596.
39. Monthioux, M.; Smith, B.; Burteaux, B.; Claye, A.; Fischer, J.; Luzzi, D., Sensitivity of single-wall carbon nanotubes to chemical processing: An electron microscopy investigation. *Carbon* 2001, *39* (8), 1251–1272.

40. Zaman, M.; Ahmad, E.; Qadeer, A.; Rabbani, G.; Khan, R. H., Nanoparticles in relation to peptide and protein aggregation. *International Journal of Nanomedicine* 2014, 9, 899–912.
41. Anzar, N.; Hasan, R.; Tyagi, M.; Yadav, N.; Narang, J., Carbon nanotube-A review on synthesis, properties and plethora of applications in the field of biomedical science. *Sensors International* 2020, *1*, 100003.
42. Odom, T. W.; Huang, J.-L.; Kim, P.; Lieber, C. M., Structure and electronic properties of carbon nanotubes. *The Journal of Physical Chemistry B* 2000, 104 (13), 2794–2809.
43. Shukla, S.; Eber, F. J.; Nagarajan, A. S.; DiFranco, N. A.; Schmidt, N.; Wen, A. M.; Eiben, S.; Twyman, R. M.; Wege, C.; Steinmetz, N. F., The impact of aspect ratio on the biodistribution and tumor homing of rigid soft-matter nanorods. *Advanced Healthcare Materials* 2015, *4* (6), 874–882.
44. Scheibel, T., Protein fibers as performance proteins: New technologies and applications. *Current Opinion in Biotechnology* 2005, 16 (4), 427–433.
45. Martin, C. R.; Kohli, P., The emerging field of nanotube biotechnology. *Nature Reviews Drug Discovery* 2003, 2 (1), 29–37.
46. Hu, H.; Bhowmik, P.; Zhao, B.; Hamon, M.; Itkis, M.; Haddon, R., Determination of the acidic sites of purified single-walled carbon nanotubes by acid–base titration. *Chemical Physics Letters* 2001, 345 (1–2), 25–28.
47. Zhao, J.; Park, H.; Han, J.; Lu, J. P., Electronic properties of carbon nanotubes with covalent sidewall functionalization. *The Journal of Physical Chemistry B* 2004, 108 (14), 4227–4230.
48. Khan, N. U.; Lin, J.; Younas, M. R.; Liu, X.; Shen, L., Synthesis of gold nanorods and their performance in the field of cancer cell imaging and photothermal therapy. *Cancer Nanotechnology* 2021, *12* (1), 1–33.
49. Kazemzadeh, H.; Mozafari, M., Adsorption, delivery, and controlled release of therapeutic molecules from MOFs. In *Metal-organic frameworks for biomedical applications*, Elsevier: 2020; pp. 297–320.
50. Liu, J.; Cao, G., Solution-based synthesis of oriented one-dimensional nanomaterials. *Annual Review of Nano Research* 2008, 287–343.
51. Turkevich, J.; Stevenson, P. C.; Hillier, J., A study of the nucleation and growth processes in the synthesis of colloidal gold. *Discussions of the Faraday Society* 1951, 11, 55–75.
52. Lin, S.-Y.; Tsai, Y.-T.; Chen, C.-C.; Lin, C.-M.; Chen, C.-H., Two-step functionalization of neutral and positively charged thiols onto citrate-stabilized Au nanoparticles. *The Journal of Physical Chemistry B* 2004, 108 (7), 2134–2139.
53. Love, J. C.; Estroff, L. A.; Kriebel, J. K.; Nuzzo, R. G.; Whitesides, G. M., Self-assembled monolayers of thiolates on metals as a form of nanotechnology. *Chemical Reviews* 2005, 105 (4), 1103–1170.
54. Yeh, Y. C.; Creran, B.; Rotello, V. M., Gold nanoparticles: Preparation, properties, and applications in bionanotechnology. *Nanoscale* 2012, *4* (6), 1871–80.
55. Li, T.; Lu, X.-M.; Zhang, M.-R.; Hu, K.; Li, Z., Peptide-based nanomaterials: Self-assembly, properties and applications. *Bioactive Materials* 2022, 11, 268–282.
56. Mondal, S.; Das, S.; Nandi, A. K., A review on recent advances in polymer and peptide hydrogels. *Soft Matter* 2020, 16 (6), 1404–1454.
57. Nezami, S.; Sadeghi, M.; Mohajerani, H., A novel pH-sensitive and magnetic starch-based nanocomposite hydrogel as a controlled drug delivery system for wound healing. *Polymer Degradation and Stability* 2020, *179*, 109255.

58. Wu, J.; Lu, Y.; Wu, Z.; Li, S.; Zhang, Q.; Chen, Z.; Jiang, J.; Lin, S.; Zhu, L.; Li, C., Two-dimensional molybdenum disulfide (MoS2) with gold nanoparticles for biosensing of explosives by optical spectroscopy. *Sensors and Actuators B: Chemical* 2018, 261, 279–287.
59. Şahin, E., *Synthesis and characterization of hydroxyapatite-alumina-zirconia biocomposites.* Izmir Institute of Technology: 2006.
60. Mammadov, R.; Tekinay, A. B.; Dana, A.; Guler, M. O., Microscopic characterization of peptide nanostructures. *Micron* 2012, *43* (2–3), 69–84.
61. Ciulla, M. G.; Fontana, F.; Lorenzi, R.; Marchini, A.; Campone, L.; Sadeghi, E.; Paleari, A.; Sattin, S.; Gelain, F., Novel self-assembling cyclic peptides with reversible supramolecular nanostructures. *Materials Chemistry Frontiers*, Royal Scoiety of Chemistry, 2023.
62. Slocik, J. M.; Naik, R. R., Probing peptide–nanomaterial interactions. *Chemical Society Reviews* 2010, 39 (9), 3454–3463.
63. Yan, C.; Pochan, D. J., Rheological properties of peptide-based hydrogels for biomedical and other applications. *Chemical Society Reviews* 2010, 39 (9), 3528–3540.
64. Castelletto, V.; Hamley, I., Methods to characterize the nanostructure and molecular organization of amphiphilic peptide assemblies. *Peptide Self-Assembly: Methods and Protocols* 2018, 1777, 3–21.
65. Denzer, B. R.; Kulchar, R. J.; Huang, R. B.; Patterson, J., Advanced methods for the characterization of supramolecular hydrogels. *Gels* 2021, *7* (4), 158.
66. Zhong, Y.; Meng, F.; Deng, C.; Zhong, Z., Ligand-directed active tumor-targeting polymeric nanoparticles for cancer chemotherapy. *Biomacromolecules* 2014, *15* (6), 1955–1969.
67. Šamec, N.; Zottel, A.; Videtič Paska, A.; Jovčevska, I., Nanomedicine and immunotherapy: A step further towards precision medicine for glioblastoma. *Molecules* 2020, *25* (3), 490.
68. Raphael, B.; Khalil, T.; Workman, V. L.; Smith, A.; Brown, C. P.; Streuli, C.; Saiani, A.; Domingos, M., 3D cell bioprinting of self-assembling peptide-based hydrogels. *Materials Letters* 2017, 190, 103–106.
69. Kar, A.; Ahamad, N.; Dewani, M.; Awasthi, L.; Patil, R.; Banerjee, R., Wearable and implantable devices for drug delivery: Applications and challenges. *Biomaterials* 2022, *283*, 121435.
70. Wang, X.; Li, Y.; Zhong, C., Amyloid-directed assembly of nanostructures and functional devices for bionanoelectronics. *Journal of Materials Chemistry B* 2015, 3 (25), 4953–4958.
71. Chen, Y.; Liang, W.; Li, Y.; Wu, Y.; Chen, Y.; Xiao, W.; Zhao, L.; Zhang, J.; Li, H., Modification, application and reaction mechanisms of nano-sized iron sulfide particles for pollutant removal from soil and water: A review. *Chemical Engineering Journal* 2019, 362, 144–159.
72. Hamley, I. W., Biocatalysts based on peptide and peptide conjugate nanostructures. *Biomacromolecules* 2021, *22* (5), 1835–1855.

4 Peptides for drug delivery with nanomaterials

4.1 INTRODUCTION TO PEPTIDE-BASED NANO DELIVERY SYSTEMS

In current years, due to their high specificity, biocompatibility, and low toxicity,[1] peptides are being investigated as a potential drug delivery technique. However, one of the major limitations in peptide-based drug delivery is the fast decomposition, systemic toxicity, and low bioavailability.[2] To overcome these limitations, nanomaterials have been extensively investigated as delivery platforms for peptides.

Nanomaterials are materials with dimensions in the nanometer range (typically between 1 and 100 nm).[3] They have distinct physical, chemical, and biological features which lend them appealing for a variety of applications, including medication administration. Nanomaterials can improve the stability and bioavailability of peptides by protecting them from degradation, prolonging their circulation time, and facilitating their uptake by target cells.[4] In the following section, we will look at the usage of nanomaterials as peptide delivery platforms and their potential uses in drug delivery.

One of the most widely used nanomaterials for peptide delivery is liposomes. Liposomes are cylindrical vessels that contain a phospholipid bilayer and are capable of carrying either hydrophilic or hydrophobic medicines, including peptides.[5] The phospholipid bilayer protects the encapsulated peptides from enzymatic decomposition and increases their stability *in vivo*. Additionally, liposomes can be engineered to target specific cells or tissues through the incorporation of ligands on their surface, such as antibodies or peptides. The use of targeted liposomes can progress toward the selectivity and efficacy of peptide-based drugs.[6]

Another promising nanomaterial for peptide delivery is polymeric nanoparticles. Polymeric nanoparticles are a collection of polymers that could encapsulate hydrophilic or hydrophobic drugs, including peptides.[7] They offer several advantages over liposomes, including greater stability and the facility to encapsulate a wider range of drugs. Additionally, polymeric nanoparticles with ligands on their surfaces can be tailored to target certain cells or tissues, including various forms of peptides or antibodies. The use of targeted polymeric nanoparticles can improve the specificity and efficacy of peptide-based drugs.[8]

In addition to liposomes and polymeric nanoparticles, other nanomaterials have been investigated for peptide delivery, including dendrimers, carbon nanotubes, and gold nanoparticles.[9] Target cells and tissues can be associated with nanocarrier systems, and they can also respond to stimuli in a carefully controlled approach to generate the desired physiological responses.[10] While dendrimers are highly branched, nanoscale polymers can be engineered to encapsulate peptides and target specific cells or tissues.[11] Dendrimer molecules have a structure that resembles a tree's branching structure. They can bind to medicines and nucleic acids and change them into active forms that may be delivered to target areas without harming healthy cells.[12] The overall molecular structures are created by the covalent conjugation of synthons to the central core, and additional drugs with various functional categories can be added to their external surfaces as capping agents. Dendrimers are classified into four types based on the functional moiety in the core and peripheral groups: polyamidoamine dendrimers, polypropyleneimine peptide dendrimers, poly(L-lysine) dendrimers, citric acid dendrimers, carbohydrate-based dendrimers, and various other functionalized and ligand-anchored dendrimers.[13]

Carbon nanotubes are cylindrical structures composed of carbon atoms that can be functionalized with peptides to target specific cells or tissues.[14] Gold nanoparticles are attractive for peptide delivery due to their biocompatibility, stability, and ability to be functionalized with peptides or other ligands.[15] Their adaptable physicochemical properties allow for the covalent and noncovalent incorporation of a variety of pharmaceutically relevant substances, as well as the rational creation of innovative candidate nanoscale constructions for drug discovery. Carbon nanotubes can be functionalized with several functional groups to transport many moieties at the same time for targeting, imaging, and therapy.[16]

The use of nanomaterials for peptide delivery has several benefits over conventional medicines delivery strategies. First, nanomaterials can protect peptides from enzymatic degradation and increase their stability *in vivo*, resulting in improved bioavailability and efficacy.[17] Recent studies have shown that lipid-based nanoparticles and biocompatible, biodegradable polymeric nanocarriers have also emerged as viable oral delivery vehicles for these biopharmaceuticals because they inhibit proteases and regulate the release of proteins.[18]

Second, nanomaterials can be engineered to target specific cells or tissues, increasing the selectivity and specificity of peptide-based drugs.[19] Targeted drug delivery has become a viable method to get around these restrictions. The term "targeted delivery" (which is additionally referred to as "molecularly targeted therapy") describes the therapeutic agent's capacity to travel selectively into the site of action following administration. Such potential outcomes are achieved by substances that specifically identify specific compounds in disease tissues, enhance therapeutic index, and minimize undesirable side effects on healthy tissues.[20]

Third, nanomaterials could encapsulate a range of drugs, including hydrophilic and hydrophobic drugs, allowing for the development of combination therapies.[21] One good example of target tumors is the monoclonal antibodies, antibody fragments, polypeptides, tiny molecules, and different ligands that have been created.[22,23] One within the most popularly used ligands in clinics for tumor targeting is antibodies. Antibodies are powerful antigen-targeting agents that can deliver anticancer medications directly to tumor areas. Slow diffusion into tumor tissue, poor *in vivo* stability, and high production costs are a few drawbacks of antibodies for beneficial usage.[24,25] On the other hand, due to their vast size, antibodies have trouble entering target tissues. By adhering to the reticuloendothelial system, they can also be toxic to the liver, bone marrow, and spleen and induce immunogenicity.[26]

The application of nanomaterials for peptide delivery has significant potential in the medical care of various disorders. Peptide-based drugs are currently being researched for the treatment of cancer and diabetes, cardiovascular disease, and infectious diseases, among others.[27] For example, peptides have been developed that can target cancer cells specifically and induce apoptosis, leading to the selective destruction of cancer cells.[28] Two general procedures were proposed: (1) inducing apoptosis through mitochondrial membrane disruption and (2) disrupting the plasma membrane via micellization or hole creation.[28,29] Additionally, peptides have been developed that can inhibit the activity of enzymes involved in the progression of cardiovascular disease,[30] such as angiotensin-converting enzyme (ACE) inhibitors, commonly used for the treatment of hypertension and heart failure.[31] Currently, peptides are considered vital tools for neurodegenerative disorders (NDs) research studies and can be further used to study the properties of misfolded proteins and/or peptides. The loss of neurons in the brain develops gradually in NDs, which ultimately causes death. Furthermore, it has been predicted that brain-related diseases including Alzheimer's disease, Parkinson's disease, Huntington's disease, and amyotrophic lateral sclerosis (ALS) are responsible for a significant number of global fatalities and disabilities (25%).[27]

Further studies have shown the loss of angiotensin-converting enzyme 2 (ACE2) elevates the possibility of developing cardiac dysfunction,[32] whereas increased ACE2 activity avoids unfavorable pathological restructuring and delays the development of heart failure (HF).[33] The loss of ACE2 may also, mechanistically, result in the activation of the cardiac Nicotinamide adenine dinucleotide phosphate (NADPH) oxidase system, an increase in superoxide generation, and the activation of matrix metalloproteinases, which can further exacerbate myocardial dysfunction and remodeling.[34] The routine of nanomaterials for the targeted delivery of peptide-based ACE inhibitors has been investigated as a potential strategy for improving their efficacy and reducing their side effects.[35] For example, one study demonstrated that the encapsulation of an ACE inhibitor in liposomes improved its bioavailability and reduced its toxicity *in* vivo.[36] Similarly, the encapsulation of an ACE inhibitor in polymeric nanoparticles improved its stability and enhanced its medical efficacy in a rat model of hypertension.[37]

Peptide-based drugs have also been investigated for the treatment of infectious diseases. For example, antimicrobial peptides (AMPs) are a class of peptides that have broad-spectrum activity against bacteria, viruses, and fungi.[38] The "barrel-stave model," "carpet model," and "toroidal-pore model" are three commonly

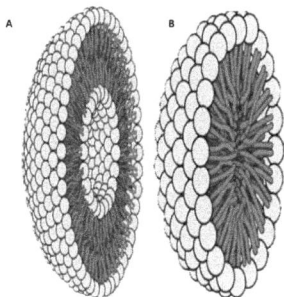

FIGURE 4.1 A schematic illustration of (A) nanomaterials bringing inherent antibacterial characteristics and (B) antimicrobial medicines/drugs based on nanoparticles. Reproduced with contend received permission from Maria C. Teixeira, *Nanomedicines for the Delivery of Antimicrobial Peptides* (AMPs); published by MDPI, 2020.

accepted hypotheses that could explain how peptide permeates the membrane of the target cell.[39] The linked peptides in the "barrel-stave model" merge to form an arrangement with a central lumen and insert into the membrane's hydrophobic core to form a transmembrane pore.[40] The "carpet model" proposes that, over a threshold concentration of membrane-bound peptide, AMPs bind to the phospholipid head covering membrane surfaces in a manner resembling carpeting and break the bilayer curvature like a detergent.[41] AMPs have several advantages over traditional antibiotics, including a lower risk of resistance development and greater selectivity for bacterial cells over host cells. However, AMPs as therapeutics have been limited use due to their limited stability and rapid degradation *in vivo*.[42]

The use of nanoparticles in AMP delivery has been investigated as a potential strategy for improving their stability and efficacy. For example, one study demonstrated that the encapsulation of an AMP in polymeric nanoparticles improved its stability and prolonged its activity against bacteria.[43] For instance, due to AMPs' vulnerability to breakdown or inactivation by pH shifts, protease activity, or high ionic strength, therapeutic usage of AMPs is constrained.[44] Additionally, AMPs can have significant hemolytic activity and low stability in blood plasma.[45] To facilitate its therapeutic usage, bioactive chemicals have been nanoencapsulated in biodegradable polymers. These biopolymers have several benefits, including site-specific delivery, protection, regulated release, increased therapeutic effectiveness, and a decrease in adverse effects. They can also shield active components from enzymatic and chemical destruction. The promising method for enhancing AMP stability and distribution is encapsulation in polymeric nanoparticles. Due to its superior biocompatibility and customizable biodegradability, poly(lactic-*co*-glycolic acid) (PLGA) nanoparticles have been used as a drug delivery device.[46,46b]

Similarly, the encapsulation of an AMP in gold nanoparticles improved its selectivity for bacterial cells over host cells and enhanced its antimicrobial activity.[47] Their significant promise in the field of nanomedicine is evidenced by their capacity to keep their structure while in circulation and their increased efficiency against germs. During early studies in this area concentrated on the potential to employ gold nanoparticles in conjunction with laser light to drastically reduce bacteria's survival through cell lysis and mechanical damage.[48]

The use of nanomaterials for peptide delivery has significantly potential for a generation of innovative therapies for a variety of ailments. Nanomaterials can improve the stability and bioavailability of peptides, allowing for the development of more effective and targeted drugs. Furthermore, the use of targeted nanomaterials can enhance the selectivity and specificity of peptide-based drugs, reducing their side effects and improving their therapeutic efficacy. As the field of nanomedicine continues to advance, the use of nanomaterials for peptide delivery will likely become increasingly important in the development of novel therapeutics for a range of diseases.

4.2 PEPTIDE-BASED NANOCARRIERS FOR DRUG DELIVERY

Peptide-based nanocarriers are emerging as a promising approach for drug delivery. These nanocarriers are composed of peptides that can self-assemble into nanostructures, such as nanoparticles, nanotubes, and nanofibers, and can encapsulate drugs within their core or on their surface.[49] Peptide-based nanocarriers have various advantages over standard drug delivery systems, including improved medication stability and bioavailability, and additionally tailored drug administration.

Peptide-based nanocarriers are constructed to be engineered to perform targeted delivery to specific cells or tissues, allowing for the selective delivery of drugs to diseased cells while minimizing toxicity to healthy cells.[50] The peptides used in these nanocarriers can be designed to bind to specific receptors on the surface of cells or to specific molecules that are overexpressed in diseased tissues. This targeted approach can improve the efficacy of drugs and reduce their side effects.[51]

Another major advantage is the ability of peptide-based nanocarriers to improve drug stability. Peptides can form stable nanostructures that protect drugs from degradation and clearance by the immune system. Furthermore, modified peptides can improve their stability, such as through the addition of chemical groups that increase their resistance to enzymatic degradation. These modifications can increase the circulation time of drugs and enhance their therapeutic effects.

Peptide-based nanocarriers can also improve drug bioavailability. The nanoscale size of these carriers allows for improved cellular uptake and penetration into tissues. Furthermore, the encapsulation of drugs within the nanocarrier can protect them from rapid metabolism and elimination, allowing for sustained release of the drug over time.

Peptide-based nanocarriers have been used for a range of therapeutic applications, including cancer therapy, cardiovascular disease, and infectious diseases. For example, peptide-based nanocarriers have been employed to deliver chemotherapeutic drugs to cancer cells, allowing for the selective delivery of the drug to cancer cells while minimizing toxicity to healthy cells. Peptide-based nanocarriers have also been used to deliver antibiotics to bacterial infections, allowing for targeted delivery of the drug to the site of infection.

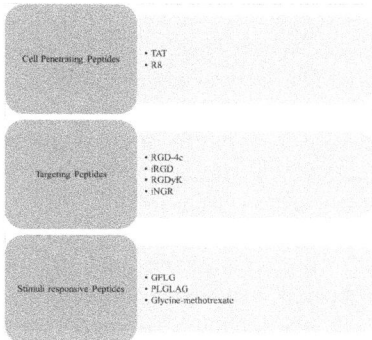

FIGURE 4.2 Classification and examples of peptide-based drug delivery systems.

One challenge in the development of peptide-based nanocarriers is their potential immunogenicity. Peptides can be recognized by the immune system as foreign, resulting in an immune reaction that can decrease the efficacy of the nanocarrier. However, this challenge can be addressed by using biocompatible and biodegradable peptides, or by modifying the peptides to reduce their immunogenicity.

4.3 APPLICATION PEPTIDE-MEDIATED DRUG DELIVERY SYSTEMS

Peptide-mediated drug transport systems are an intriguing technique for delivering targeted drugs. As peptides are short sequences of amino acid blocks that can be designed to specifically bind to target cells or tissues, peptides can be easily synthesized, modified, and functionalized, making them an attractive option for drug delivery applications.

Peptides have various advantages over conventional medication delivery systems for focused drug distribution. Peptides can be designed to specifically target diseased cells or tissues, allowing for the delivery of medicines directly towards the site of action.[52] This can reduce the dose required to achieve therapeutic effects, minimizing side effects and toxicity. Peptides can also increase drug stability, solubility, and bioavailability, allowing for improved drug delivery and efficacy.[53] Physiological barriers, biochemical difficulties in identifying and validating molecular targets, and pharmacological difficulties in developing effective methods of conjugating targeting ligands to nanosystems are the main obstacles to therapeutic targeting. The difficulty with drug targeting is not only getting the drug to an appropriate place but also retaining it there for a suitable length of time to cause pharmacological effects. The vascular endothelium and basement membrane serve as the initial and most important barriers for an intravenously delivered nanosystem.[54]

Peptides can be discovered in a wide range of drug delivery methods, such as nanoparticles, liposomes, and hydrogels. Peptide-based nanoparticles can be engineered to specifically target diseased cells or tissues, allowing medications to be transported directly to the site of infection.[55] Peptide-based liposomes can be used to improve drug stability and bioavailability and can be modified to enhance their targeting capabilities. While the majority of protein/peptide-based medications are still provided parenterally, the pharmaceutical industry is under enormous pressure to create oral delivery systems that will improve patient acceptability and convenience.[6]

Peptide-based hydrogels can be used for sustained drug release, allowing for long-term drug delivery.[56] The three-dimensional (3D) network's porous microstructure is created by physically or chemically cross-linking synthetic, organic, or hybrid polymers. Even though synthetic polymers have better mechanical properties, protein- and peptide-based hydrogels are becoming more popular because they are more biocompatible and have more adaptable properties.[57] The ability of protein- and peptide-based hydrogels to react to environmental cues including temperature, pH, light, and tiny molecules makes them a potential class of biomaterials. A potent method of medicine delivery that takes advantage of the special properties of the target organ infection is an inflammation-targeting hydrogel. A more effective and secure method of administering medications locally at the site of inflammation with little exposure to nearby healthy tissues is through the use of hydrogels that target inflammation.[58]

One example of peptide-mediated drug delivery application is the use of cyclic RGD (arginine-glycine-aspartic acid) peptides for the targeted delivery of anticancer drugs.[59] The RGD peptide family is regarded as arguably the most significant ligand for integrin receptors' extracellular domain. Due to the specific expression of these receptors in various human body tissues and the close relationship between their expression profile and varied pathophysiological circumstances- their condition was ideal targets for the diagnosis and therapy of many diseases as well as the regeneration of various organs.[60] Furthermore, cyclic RGD peptides are designed to bind particularly to integrin receptors excessively expressed on the outermost layer of cancer cells.[61] When coupled to an anticancer drug, cyclic RGD peptides can selectively deliver the drug to cancer cells, minimizing toxicity to healthy cells. This approach is effective in preclinical studies, and multiple clinical studies are currently being conducted.

Another example of peptide-mediated drug delivery application is the use of cell-penetrating peptides (CPPs) for the delivery of therapeutic molecules into cells.[62] CPPs, often referred to as protein transduction domains (PTDs), are a unique method for delivering big particles and macromolecules that pass across biological membranes and tissue barriers. This method was developed to circumvent the cell membrane impermeability. CPPs are cationic or amphipathic peptides that are water soluble, relatively short (up to 30 amino acids in length), and capable of transporting large macromolecules through cellular membranes.[63] They are short peptides that can facilitate the uptake of molecules into cells, including proteins, nucleic acids, and small molecules. CPPs can be utilized to transfer a range of therapeutics, including anticancer drugs, gene therapies, and vaccines.[64]

Peptide-mediated drug delivery systems also have the ability to take precedence over some of the boundaries of the conventional system of drug supply methods, such as poor solubility, instability, and low bioavailability, which will be further discussed in the chapter. Peptides can be designed to improve drug solubility, stability, and bioavailability, allowing for improved drug delivery and efficacy. Furthermore, peptides can be modified to enhance their specificity and selectivity, minimizing side effects and toxicity. Also, the capacity of the active ingredient to penetrate the skin in sufficient amounts to produce the intended therapeutic effects greatly influences topical drug delivery. The primary barrier to transdermal absorption is the stratum corneum, which is the outermost layer of skin. Extracellular lipids like ceramides, cholesterol, and free fatty acids in this layer combine with cellular components in the cornified layer of the intrafollicular epidermis to produce complexes that act as strong resistance to microbial invasion and desiccation.[65] We understand that to reduce the impermeability of the cell membrane peptide-mediated drug delivery is a successful tool to be used.

Hence, we understand that the application of various forms of peptide-mediated is a promising option for tailored medicine delivery mediated through drug delivery systems. Peptides can be designed to specifically target diseased cells or tissues, allowing for the delivery of drugs directly to the site of action. Peptides can also increase drug stability, solubility, and bioavailability, allowing for improved drug transport and efficiency. As the field of peptide-mediated drug delivery continues to advance, this approach will likely become increasingly important in the development of novel therapeutics for a range of diseases.

Peptides are used for drug delivery and can be classified as shown in Figure 4.2. Let us know each of the peptides and their mechanisms in detail.

4.4 CPPS FOR DRUG DELIVERY

CPPs are a type of small-sized peptides that can aid in the absorption of a variety of substances, including proteins, nucleic acids, and small molecules, into cells.[66] The first sequence reported to be capable of traversing cell membranes and gaining intracellular access was the human immunodeficiency virus type 1 (HIV-1)-encoded transactivator of transcription (Tat) peptide,[67] which led to the discovery of this new class of peptides in 1988. This discovery was followed a short time later by the use of penetration to deliver a tiny exogenous peptide. Later research revealed that these peptides' short domains are frequently in charge of cellular absorption.[68] Therefore, compared to the initial Tat peptide, these translocation sequences might be reduced to a limited amino acid without losing their ability to penetrate cells.[63,67]

Tat, polyarginine, penetrating, transportan, and Pep-1 (Table 4.1) are among the most often utilized peptides in CPP, while the choice of CPP frequently relies on the type of application.

TABLE 4.1
Examples of synthetic CPPs with their sequences

Name	Sequence
Tat	GRKKRRQRRRPPQ
Penetratin	RQIKIWFQNRRMKWKK
Transportan	GWTLNSAGYLLGKINLKALAALAKKIL
Pep-1	KETWWETWWTEWSQPKKKRKV

CPPs can be utilized to deliver medicines, including anticancer drugs, gene therapies,[69] and vaccines. CPPs can enhance drug bioavailability and efficacy by improving cellular transport uptake, reducing their dose and toxicity, and targeting specific cells or tissues.[62]

4.4.1 Mechanisms of CPP

The mechanisms underlying CPP-mediated cellular uptake are not completely understood, but it is believed to involve complex formation between CPPs and cargo molecules, which are subsequently picked up by cells via endocytosis or other mechanisms.[70] CPPs can interact with a variety of cellular structures, including the plasma membrane, cytoplasmic vesicles, and nuclear envelope, allowing for the efficient delivery of cargo molecules to intracellular targets.

CPP and cargo can be joined in one of two ways. In the initial strategy, the CPP/cargo sequences are produced in *Escherichia coli*, followed by the purification of the recombinant fusion protein.[71] The second method entails creating a complex by connecting CPP and cargo. The majority of the suggested CPPs, including Tat,[72] Poly-Arg,[73] transportan,[74] and penetratin,[71] are cells ingest payloads that are covalently bound to them. Although a variety of cargoes have been delivered using these covalent bonds effectively, they do have significant drawbacks.

CPPs are typically small, cationic peptides that are rich in arginine and/or lysine residues.[75] Examples of CPPs include the well-known Tat peptide, derived from the HIV-1 Tat protein, and the Antennapedia peptide, derived from the *Drosophila melanogaster* Antennapedia homeodomain protein.[76] CPPs can be synthesized as examples shown in Table 4.1, by chemical methods or recombinant Nicotinamide adenine dinucleotide phosphate (DNA) technology, and can be considerably optimized in terms of stability, specificity, and efficacy (Table 4.2).

CPPs have several advantages over traditional drug delivery methods. CPP-mediated drug delivery is a noninvasive, versatile approach that can be used for a wide range of therapeutic molecules, including those that are difficult to deliver by other means.[78] CPPs can be modified to target specific cell types or tissues, allowing for the targeted administration of medicines to sick cells or tissues. Furthermore, CPP-mediated drug delivery can improve the bioavailability and efficacy of drugs, reducing their dose and toxicity.[79]

TABLE 4.2
CPP-cargo conjugate updates for delivery through the plasma membrane[77]

Imaging	Nucleic acid delivery	Protein delivery	Therapeutics
Quantum dots	siRNA	Antibodies	Small molecule drugs
Fluorophores	DNA	Proteins	Peptide-based drugs
Radiolabels	RNA		
Magnetic resonance imaging (MRI) contrast agents	Peptide Nucleic Acid (PNA)		

CPP-mediated drug delivery has been used for a range of therapeutic applications. For example, CPPs have been used for the delivery of small interfering RNA (siRNA) for gene silencing, and for the delivery of peptides and proteins for the treatment of a variety of ailments such as cancer diabetes and cardiovascular disease.[80] CPP-mediated drug delivery has also been used for the delivery of imaging agents, allowing for the visualization of specific cells or tissues.[81] A study on quantum dots (QDs) showed that QD-fluorescent protein complexes by cells depended on the presence of CPP within the QD-protein combinations. Once inside the cells, these QD complexes were mostly located within endolysosomal compartments, demonstrating that their entry into cells was primarily through endocytosis, a cellular process. An alternative method, cellular microinjection, was also employed to deliver the QD-fluorescent protein complexes directly into cells, bypassing the endocytic pathway.[82]

One limitation of CPP-mediated drug delivery is that the uptake of cargo molecules can be inefficient and can vary depending on the cell type, concentration, and modification of the CPPs.[83] Additionally, the use of CPPs for drug delivery can be limited by potential toxicity and immunogenicity concerns.[62] However, these limitations can be overcome by optimizing the design and modification of CPPs, as well as by careful selection of cargo molecules.

CPP-mediated drug delivery is a potential strategy for focused distribution of therapeutics to cells and tissues. CPPs can facilitate the uptake of a range of molecules, allowing for the delivery of drugs that are difficult to deliver by other means. CPP-mediated drug delivery may enhance drug bioavailability and effectiveness, reducing their dose and toxicity. As the field of CPP-mediated drug delivery continues to advance, this approach will likely become increasingly important in the development of novel therapeutics for a range of diseases.

4.5 TARGETED DRUG DELIVERY USING PEPTIDES

Paul Ehrlich was the first to propose the theory of targeted drug administration around the turn of the 20th century. The idea was inspired by the discovery that diseased tissue contains a variety of intricate cellular and noncellular components, some of which could be addressed by drugs that function as "magic bullets," selectively eradicating diseased cells without harming healthy ones. This would increase the effectiveness of medications and lessen their side effects.[84,85]

Generally, targeted drug delivery uses either active or passive target mechanisms. Due to intrinsic drug delivery system characteristics like size, shape, and charge as well as unique characteristics of the addressed areas such as local vasculature and lymphatic drainage, medicines concentrate at sick sites in passive targeting. For instance, at tumor locations, the lymphatic drainage is either absent or severely compromised, and the adjacent vasculature is leaky. Under these circumstances, drug delivery systems exhibit what is known as the increased permeability and retention effect, which permits the tumor tissue to preferentially accumulate high molecular weight polymers as well as nanoscale particles with a diameter of roughly 20–500 nm.[86] In turn, receptor-directed active targeting is accomplished by affixing ligands that bind to specific receptors on the medication or drug carrier. Due to their intrinsic affinity for several bodily receptors, peptides have emerged as one of the most widely employed targeting agents in drug delivery. As a consequence of tumor-specific marker overexpression, targeting peptides most often serve as a delivery method for distinct tumor cells or tissues.[87]

Peptide-targeted drug delivery is a potential strategy for the treatment of a variety of disorders, including cancer, cardiovascular disease, and neurodegenerative disorders.[88] This approach involves the application of peptides to specifically target cells or tissues and permits drug distribution on a case-by-case basis to diseased cells while minimizing toxicity to healthy cells. One such example is that although the effectiveness of the majority of these treatments is lacking, recent efforts of the strategies were developed in order to triumph over the obstacles encountered during successful treatment, including changes in the blood-brain barrier's (BBB) permeability efficiency and carrier and receptor-mediated drug transport. To help in drug distribution across BBB, several techniques include lipidization of a molecule with a lipid layer, disruption of BBB using ultrasonic technology or radiation therapy, and usage of nanomaterials.[89,90]

Peptides can be engineered to specifically target cells or tissues by exploiting various mechanisms, such as receptor-mediated targeting, enzymatic targeting, and affinity targeting.[91] Receptor-mediated use of peptides that bind to specific receptors on the surface of cells is known as targeting, allowing for the selective uptake of drugs by those cells. Enzymatic targeting involves the use of peptides that are cleaved by enzymes that are specifically expressed by diseased cells, releasing the drug in a targeted manner.[52] It is incredibly promising to use changed enzyme activity and expression for diagnostics, medication targeting, and drug release.[92] Affinity targeting involves the use of peptides that bind to specific molecules that are specifically expressed by diseased cells, enabling the targeted delivery of medicines to certain cells.[93]

Using peptides for targeted medicine delivery has several benefits over conventional drug delivery techniques. Peptide-mediated drug delivery could enhance the specificity and efficacy of drugs, reducing the dose and toxicity required for therapeutic effects. Furthermore, targeted drug delivery could enhance drug bioavailability and circulation time, enhancing their therapeutic effects.[94] Nevertheless, the fundamental benefit of using macromolecules as drug delivery agents is their cellular internalization mechanism(s). Although complexes greater than 1 kDa are naturally impermeable to cell membranes, cells have a number of active internalization mechanisms that allow the cellular entry of large molecular complexes. This process, known as endocytosis, involves the cell membrane puncturing to engulf molecules and external fluid in an intracellular membrane-bound vesicle, or endosome, which will then migrate within the cell membrane.[93]

Targeted drug delivery using peptides is applied for a range of therapeutic applications. For example, peptides have been used to target cancer cells, permitting the selective and targeted delivery of chemotherapeutic drugs to those cells while minimizing toxicity to healthy cells. Nanoparticles can increase the intracellular concentration of medicines in cancer cells while minimizing damage to normal cells by employing combined passive and active targeting techniques.[95] Additionally, when nanoparticles bind to particular receptors and then enter the cell, they are typically engulfed by endosomes by receptor-mediated endocytosis, avoiding identification of P-glycoprotein, one of the primary drug resistance mechanisms.[95] Despite nanoparticles are effective drug delivery vehicles, a number of difficulties remain, including inadequate oral bioavailability, circulatory instability, insufficient tissue distribution, and cytotoxicity.[96] Peptides have also been used to target inflamed tissues in autoimmune diseases, allowing for the selective delivery of anti-inflammatory drugs to those tissues.[96] Asthma, chronic obstructive pulmonary disease, osteoarthritis, rheumatoid arthritis, inflammatory bowel diseases (ulcerative colitis, Crohn's disease), celiac disease, autoinflammatory syndrome, and inflammation associated with transplantation are a few examples of diseases for which the application of targeted drug delivery with nanosystems. Hence, chronic inflammatory disordersis considered as one of the most frequent causes of death and a major decrement in quality of life due to toxicity and insufficient tissue dispersion.[97]

While the benefits of targeted drug delivery are high, there are a few limitations as well. One challenge The stability and specificity of the peptides are important considerations in the development of peptide-mediated drug delivery systems.[98] Peptides can be degraded by enzymes and cleared by the immune system, reducing their efficacy and specificity.[99] However, peptide stability can be improved by chemical modifications or by the use of nanomaterials, such as liposomes or nanoparticles, which can preserve peptides from degradation and improve their performance circulation time as discussed in earlier chapters.

In conclusion, we understand that targeted drug delivery using peptides is a potential method for treating many disorders. Peptides can be engineered to specifically target cells or tissues, permitting drug distribution on a case-by-case basis to diseased cells while minimizing toxicity to healthy cells. As the field of peptide-mediated drug delivery continues to advance, this approach will likely become increasingly important in the discovery of innovative medicines for a variety of disorders.

4.6 STIMULI-RESPONSIVE PEPTIDES

The capacity of DDSs to change their modification as a result of certain triggers is known as stimuli-responsiveness. The ability of smart DDSs to function precisely and under control in order to lessen the severity of unwanted effects and increase the therapeutic efficiency of medications is a crucial characteristic of these systems. The features of DDSs can be greatly altered by a variety of stimulation agents, including pH, light, magnetic fields, and enzymes, by regulating their permeability, internalization, size reductions, and drug release.[100] Stimuli-responsive systems can be manually activated by external effects that are photothermal, magnetic, electric, or acoustic as well as in reaction to local environmental parameters like pH, temperature, redox state, and the concentration of particular molecules (such as O_2, urea, and enzymes).[101]

The small sequence of amino acids are the foundation blocks of proteins that known as stimulus-responsive peptides and have the capacity to change their shape or behave differently in response to stimuli from the outside world. This activity is a result of the interactions and inherent properties of the amino acids that provide base to the peptide chain. The sequence of amino acids can be carefully planned by researchers to create peptides that react to particular triggers.[102]

One of the most exciting aspects of stimuli-responsive peptides lies in their potential to revolutionize drug delivery. Traditional drug delivery systems often lack precision and control, leading to unintended side effects and reduced therapeutic efficacy. Stimuli-responsive peptides offer a solution by enabling targeted drug release at the site of action. For instance, peptides are designed to remain stable during circulation but undergo conformational changes in response to specific conditions present in disease sites, such as the slightly acidic environment of tumors.[103] This enables the controlled release of therapeutic agents precisely where they are needed, minimizing damage to healthy tissues.

In tissue engineering, stimuli-responsive peptides are being employed to create scaffolds that mimic the extracellular matrix, providing support and cues for cells to grow and differentiate. These peptides can change their properties in response to signals from surrounding cells, enhancing tissue regeneration and repair. Peptidases are hydrolase-class enzymes that use water to dissociate covalent peptide bonds (>C(=O)NH-R). There have been reports of a wide range of peptidases accumulating more commonly at lesion sites such as tumor sites and ischemia regions. The classes of those peptidases can be divided into metallo- (e.g., gelatinases, matrilysins), cysteine- (e.g., cathepsin B, cathepsin C), serine- (e.g., urokinase (uPA), pseudoaneurysm (PSA) , thrombin), threonine- (e.g., testes-specific protease 50, threonine aspartase 1), and aspartic proteases (e.g., cathepsin D, cathepsin E, memapsin).[104] As a result, scientists are now interested in utilizing these characteristics of tumor tissues to create biocompatible, peptidase-responsive DDSs. Additionally, they can be used to create "smart" materials that change their mechanical properties or surface characteristics in response to environmental changes. This opens up new avenues for designing adaptive materials for applications in robotics, sensors, and beyond.[105]

While stimuli-responsive peptides have garnered significant attention in the biomedical field, their potential extends far beyond healthcare. In materials science, these peptides are being harnessed to create coatings that can prevent biofouling by responding to changes in the surrounding environment. They also play a role in controlled release systems for agricultural applications, enabling the precise delivery of nutrients or pesticides to crops.[106]

Despite the immense potential of stimuli-responsive peptides, there are challenges that researchers are actively addressing. Designing peptides with the desired responsiveness while maintaining stability and safety is a complex task. One method for increasing medication efficiency is the use of smart DDSs. There are many different peptidase-responsive peptides utilized in DDSs, but a few have drawn special attention because of their exceptional efficacy (Figure 4.1). One of these peptides is the GFLG (Gly-Phe-Leu-Gly) tetrapeptide, which can be broken down by the cysteine protease cathepsin B, which is expressed at higher levels in most types of tumors than in healthy tissue.[107] The use of GFLG in a DDS has been reported by Zhang and colleagues. The system that they created consists of cathepsin B-cleavable GFLG that has been PEGylated lysine dendrimer nanoparticles that have been coupled with gemcitabine. The dendrimer is highly biodegradable and water-soluble due to its construction from the amino acid residue. In turn, PEGylation increases the system's solubility and reduces immunogenicity, and when combined with the dendrimer's branched architecture, it enables an extended blood circulation period of the medication, allowing for less frequent dosing. When cathepsin B cleaves the GFLG, the DDS is intended to release gemcitabine. According to the investigations, the gemcitabine release was more than 80% higher in the cathepsin B environment (*in vitro*) in comparison with the control environment. In a 4T1 mouse breast cancer model, the nanoparticles revealed a relative tumor suppression volume of 82 ± 38%, with no indication of harm to normal cells, demonstrating the system's high biocompatibility and, in particular, the effectiveness of GFLG. The drug release kinetics showed that 60% of loaded gemcitabine was released within 30 min, while was discharged 90% of the drug was released in 24 h.[108,109]

Additionally, the translation of these concepts from the lab to real-world applications requires rigorous testing, optimization, and regulatory considerations. The future of stimuli-responsive peptides is poised for exciting advancements. As our understanding of peptide chemistry, molecular interactions, and cellular processes deepens, we can expect to see even more sophisticated designs that cater to a wide range of stimuli and applications. Collaborations between scientists, engineers, and medical experts will be crucial in realizing the full potential of these peptides in addressing pressing global challenges.

With their ability to intelligently respond to external triggers, these peptides hold promise for transforming industries and improving the quality of life. As research progresses and technologies mature, we can anticipate a future where stimuli-responsive peptides play an integral role in personalized medicine, advanced materials, and cutting-edge biotechnologies, pushing the boundaries of what is possible at the interface of nature and innovation.

4.7 AMPS AND ANTICANCER PEPTIDES

Anticancer peptides (ACPs), also known as a type of CPPs with anticancer properties, are a diverse group of small peptides that exhibit cytotoxic effects specifically against cancer cells while sparing healthy cells.[110] Peptides can be grouped generally into multiple groups based on their origins, structures, and mechanisms of action.

ACPs exert their anticancer effects through mainly three types of mechanisms: (1) apoptosis induction, where many ACPs trigger programmed cell death (apoptosis) in cancer cells by disrupting the balance between pro-apoptotic and anti-apoptotic factors; (2) cell cycle arrest, where some ACPs interfere with the cell cycle progression of cancer cells, leading to cell cycle arrest and subsequent cell death; and (3) inhibition of angiogenesis, where ACPs can inhibit the formation of new blood vessels (angiogenesis), a crucial process for tumor growth.[111,112]

There are several ACPs which have gained recognition for their anticancer potential. Magainin-derived peptides are one such example where magainins and their derivatives have demonstrated selective cytotoxicity towards cancer cells, making them promising candidates for cancer therapy. Another example is Pepstatin A, which is originally an aspartic protease inhibitor. Pepstatin A has shown promise as an ACP by inhibiting the proliferation of certain cancer cell lines.[113]

Despite the development of ACPs into effective cancer therapeutics, ACP comes with its share of challenges, including issues related to stability, specificity, and delivery as discussed previously. Hence, it is required to research further to focus on improving these aspects and expanding the repertoire of ACPs for a broader range of cancers, such as the help of nanocomposites to overcome such limitations of ACPs.

Another important form of therapeutic peptides is AMPs, also referred to as host defense peptides. These are a diverse group of short peptides found in various organisms, including humans, plants, and animals.[114] They serve as a first line of defense against microbial infections and can be categorized based on their structures and mechanisms of action. Their mechanisms of action (Figure 4.3) include a range of mechanisms to combat microorganisms, such as (1) membrane disruption, which is the most common way to disrupt the integrity of microbial cell membranes, causing leakage of cellular contents and cell death; (2) inhibition of cell wall synthesis, which is present in some AMPs that interfere with the synthesis of bacterial cell walls, weakening the structural integrity of the microorganism; and (3) immunomodulatory effects, where the AMPs believe to alter the host immunological response, improving the body's ability to fight infections.[115,116]

As ACPs numerous AMPs have been discovered and researched for their antimicrobial properties: LL-37, derived from human cathelicidin, is a 37-residue, amphipathic, helical peptide found all over the body and has been demonstrated to have a broad spectrum of antibacterial properties and immunomodulatory effects.[117] Next is the Nisin, a well-known bacteriocin produced by certain lactic acid bacteria and used as a food preservative due to its antimicrobial properties.[118]

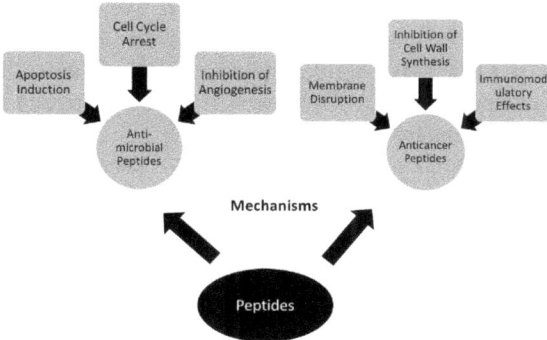

FIGURE 4.3 Summary and description of the mode of action of AMPs as well as ACPs.

Many AMPs work as ACPs as well. For example, melittin is a peptide derived from bee venom with antibacterial and anticancer characteristics that promote cancer cell hemolysis, but when taken intravenously can cause severe allergic adverse effects.[119]

Despite their effectiveness, challenges such as susceptibility to proteolytic degradation and limited specificity against certain pathogens exist in the development of AMP-based therapies. Research is ongoing to optimize AMPs for clinical use and mitigate these challenges.

Both AMPs and ACPs serve as a foundation for understanding the unique properties and potential applications of these important peptide groups in the field of oncology and infectious disease treatment.

4.8 CHALLENGES AND PROSPECTS OF PEPTIDE-BASED DRUG DELIVERY

While peptide-based drug delivery has shown great promise, there are still several challenges that must be solved in order to completely realize their potential. Some of these challenges include:

1. **Stability:** Peptides are susceptible to degradation by enzymes and are rapidly cleared from the body, which can limit their therapeutic efficacy. Researchers are developing ways to improve the stability of peptides by modifying them with protective groups or by designing peptides that are less prone to degradation.[120]
2. **Immunogenicity:** As mentioned earlier, peptides can be recognized by the immune system as foreign, resulting in an immunological response that can impair the efficiency of the peptide-based drug delivery method. Researchers are working to develop strategies to reduce the immunogenicity of peptides by modifying their structures or by using biocompatible and biodegradable peptides.[121]

3. Specificity: Peptide-based drug delivery systems need to be highly specifically targeted to target diseased cells while minimizing toxicity to healthy cells. Designing peptides that specifically bind to diseased cells or tissues can be challenging and necessitates an in-depth knowledge of the disease's fundamental biology.[122]
4. Manufacturing: Peptide-based drug delivery systems can be difficult to produce on a vast scale. Developing efficient and cost-effective methods for producing peptide-based nanocarriers is an ongoing challenge.[122]

Despite these challenges, the future of peptide-based drug delivery looks bright. Technological advances in peptide synthesis, nanotechnology, and imaging techniques are creating new opportunities for targeted medication delivery. Some of the prospects of peptide-based drug delivery include:

1. Personalized medicine: Peptide-based drug delivery systems can be tailored to specific patients based on their genetic and molecular profiles. This could lead to more effective treatments that are better tolerated by patients.[123]
2. Combination therapies: Peptide-based drug delivery systems can be used to deliver multiple drugs simultaneously to target different aspects of a disease. This could lead to more effective treatments and fewer side effects.[124]
3. Regenerative medicine: Peptide-based nanocarriers can be used to deliver growth factors and other molecules that promote tissue regeneration. This could lead to new treatments for conditions such as heart disease and spinal cord injuries.[125]
4. Imaging and diagnostics: Peptides are employed to detect imaging agents and visualize diseased cells or tissues. This could lead to earlier diagnosis and more targeted treatments.[16]

In conclusion, we can say that peptide-based drug delivery has the promise for revolutionary change in the medical industry. While there are still challenges that need to be addressed, ongoing research is paving the way for new and innovative peptide-based drug delivery systems that could lead to more effective and personalized treatments for a wide range of diseases.

A. PRACTICAL QUESTIONS

1. How do peptides enhance the effectiveness of drug delivery when combined with nanomaterials?
2. What are the key advantages of using peptides as carriers for drug delivery compared to traditional methods?
3. Can you explain the role of nanomaterials in optimizing the targeted delivery of therapeutic agents using peptides?

4. What are some examples of stimuli-responsive peptides that have been successfully employed in nanomaterial-based drug delivery systems, and how do they work?
5. How do researchers address challenges related to the stability, biocompatibility, and controlled release of drugs when developing peptide-nanomaterial hybrid systems for drug delivery?

REFERENCES

1. Drayton, M.; Kizhakkedathu, J. N.; Straus, S. K., Towards robust delivery of antimicrobial peptides to combat bacterial resistance. *Molecules* 2020, *25* (13), 3048.
2. Haney, E. F.; Straus, S. K.; Hancock, R. E., Reassessing the host defense peptide landscape. *Frontiers in Chemistry* 2019, , 7, 435645.
3. Asha, A. B.; Narain, R., Nanomaterials properties. In *Polymer science and nanotechnology*, Elsevier: 2020; pp. 343–359.
4. Kreyling, W. G.; Semmler-Behnke, M.; Chaudhry, Q., A complementary definition of nanomaterial. *Nano Today* 2010, 5 (3), 165–168.
5. van der Koog, L.; Gandek, T. B.; Nagelkerke, A., Liposomes and extracellular vesicles as drug delivery systems: A comparison of composition, pharmacokinetics, and functionalization. *Advanced Healthcare Materials* 2022, *11* (5), 2100639.
6. Jash, A.; Ubeyitogullari, A.; Rizvi, S. S., Liposomes for oral delivery of protein and peptide-based therapeutics: Challenges, formulation strategies, and advances. *Journal of Materials Chemistry B* 2021, 9 (24), 4773–4792.
7. Pagels, R. F.; Prud'Homme, R. K., Polymeric nanoparticles and microparticles for the delivery of peptides, biologics, and soluble therapeutics. *Journal of Controlled Release* 2015, 219, 519–535.
8. Akagi, T.; Baba, M.; Akashi, M., Preparation of nanoparticles by the self-organization of polymers consisting of hydrophobic and hydrophilic segments: Potential applications. *Polymer* 2007, *48* (23), 6729–6747.
9. Kesharwani, P.; Gothwal, A.; Iyer, A. K.; Jain, K.; Chourasia, M. K.; Gupta, U., Dendrimer nanohybrid carrier systems: An expanding horizon for targeted drug and gene delivery. *Drug Discovery Today* 2018, 23 (2), 300–314.
10. Bharali, D. J.; Khalil, M.; Gurbuz, M.; Simone, T. M.; Mousa, S. A., Nanoparticles and cancer therapy: A concise review with emphasis on dendrimers. *International Journal of Nanomedicine* 2009, 4, 1–7.
11. Kannan, R.; Nance, E.; Kannan, S.; Tomalia, D. A., Emerging concepts in dendrimer-based nanomedicine: From design principles to clinical applications. *Journal of Internal Medicine* 2014, 276 (6), 579–617.
12. Kesharwani, P.; Jain, K.; Jain, N. K., Dendrimer as nanocarrier for drug delivery. *Progress in Polymer Science* 2014, *39* (2), 268–307.
13. Dey, A. D.; Bigham, A.; Esmaeili, Y.; Ashrafizadeh, M.; Moghaddam, F. D.; Tan, S. C.; Yousefiasl, S.; Sharma, S.; Maleki, A.; Rabiee, N.; Kumar, A. P.; Thakur, V. K.; Orive, G.; Sharifi, E.; Kumar, A.; Makvandi, P., Dendrimers as nanoscale vectors: Unlocking the bars of cancer therapy. *Seminars in Cancer Biology* 2022, 86, 396–419.
14. Raphey, V. R.; Henna, T. K.; Nivitha, K. P.; Mufeedha, P.; Sabu, C.; Pramod, K., Advanced biomedical applications of carbon nanotube. *Materials Science and Engineering: C* 2019, 100, 616–630.
15. Amina, S. J.; Guo, B., A review on the synthesis and functionalization of gold nanoparticles as a drug delivery vehicle. *International Journal of Nanomedicine* 2020, 15, 9823–9857.

16. Prato, M.; Kostarelos, K.; Bianco, A., Functionalized carbon nanotubes in drug design and discovery. *Accounts of Chemical Research* 2008, 41 (1), 60–68.
17. Ibrahim, Y. H. Y.; Regdon, G.; Hamedelniel, E. I.; Sovány, T., Review of recently used techniques and materials to improve the efficiency of orally administered proteins/peptides. *DARU Journal of Pharmaceutical Sciences* 2020, 28, 403–416.
18. Santalices, I.; Gonella, A.; Torres, D.; Alonso, M. J., Advances on the formulation of proteins using nanotechnologies. *Journal of Drug Delivery Science and Technology* 2017, 42, 155–180.
19. Araste, F.; Abnous, K.; Hashemi, M.; Taghdisi, S. M.; Ramezani, M.; Alibolandi, M., Peptide-based targeted therapeutics: Focus on cancer treatment. *Journal of Controlled Release* 2018, 292, 141–162.
20. Tsuji, A., Small molecular drug transfer across the blood-brain barrier via carrier-mediated transport systems. *NeuroRX* 2005, 2 (1), 54–62.
21. Acar, H.; Srivastava, S.; Chung, E. J.; Schnorenberg, M. R.; Barrett, J. C.; LaBelle, J. L.; Tirrell, M., Self-assembling peptide-based building blocks in medical applications. *Advanced Drug Delivery Reviews* 2017, 110, 65–79.
22. Karami Fath, M.; Babakhaniyan, K.; Zokaei, M.; Yaghoubian, A.; Akbari, S.; Khorsandi, M.; Soofi, A.; Nabi-Afjadi, M.; Zalpoor, H.; Jalalifar, F., Anti-cancer peptide-based therapeutic strategies in solid tumors. *Cellular & Molecular Biology Letters* 2022, 27 (1), 33.
23. Senapati, S.; Mahanta, A. K.; Kumar, S.; Maiti, P., Controlled drug delivery vehicles for cancer treatment and their performance. *Signal Transduction and Targeted Therapy* 2018, 3 (1), 7.
24. Mohit, E.; Hashemi, A.; Allahyari, M., Breast cancer immunotherapy: Monoclonal antibodies and peptide-based vaccines. *Expert Review of Clinical Immunology* 2014, 10 (7), 927–961.
25. Rahman, M.; Ahmad, M. Z.; Kazmi, I.; Akhter, S.; Afzal, M.; Gupta, G.; Jalees Ahmed, F.; Anwar, F., Advancement in multifunctional nanoparticles for the effective treatment of cancer. *Expert Opinion on Drug Delivery* 2012, 9 (4), 367–381.
26. Liu, R.; Li, X.; Xiao, W.; Lam, K. S., Tumor-targeting peptides from combinatorial libraries. *Advanced Drug Delivery Reviews* 2017, 110, 13–37.
27. Baig, M. H.; Ahmad, K.; Saeed, M.; Alharbi, A. M.; Barreto, G. E.; Ashraf, G. M.; Choi, I., Peptide based therapeutics and their use for the treatment of neurodegenerative and other diseases. *Biomedicine & Pharmacotherapy* 2018, 103, 574–581.
28. Papo, N.; Shai, Y., Host defense peptides as new weapons in cancer treatment. *Cellular and Molecular Life Sciences CMLS* 2005, 62, 784–790.
29. Sato, A. K.; Viswanathan, M.; Kent, R. B.; Wood, C. R., Therapeutic peptides: Technological advances driving peptides into development. *Current Opinion in Biotechnology* 2006, 17 (6), 638–642.
30. Phelan, M.; Kerins, D., The potential role of milk-derived peptides in cardiovascular disease. *Food & Function* 2011, 2 (3–4), 153–167.
31. De Leo, F.; Panarese, S.; Gallerani, R.; Ceci, L., Angiotensin converting enzyme (ACE) inhibitory peptides: Production and implementation of functional food. *Current Pharmaceutical Design* 2009, 15 (31), 3622–3643.
32. Chamsi-Pasha, M. A.; Shao, Z.; Tang, W. W., Angiotensin-converting enzyme 2 as a therapeutic target for heart failure. *Current Heart Failure Reports* 2014, 11, 58–63.
33. Tikellis, C.; Bernardi, S.; Burns, W. C., Angiotensin-converting enzyme 2 is a key modulator of the renin–angiotensin system in cardiovascular and renal disease. *Current Opinion in Nephrology and Hypertension* 2011, 20 (1), 62–68.

34. Bodiga, S.; Zhong, J. C.; Wang, W.; Basu, R.; Lo, J.; Liu, G. C.; Guo, D.; Holland, S. M.; Scholey, J. W.; Penninger, J. M., Enhanced susceptibility to biomechanical stress in ACE2 null mice is prevented by loss of the p47phox NADPH oxidase subunit. *Cardiovascular Research* 2011, 91 (1), 151–161.
35. Bertrand, N.; Wu, J.; Xu, X.; Kamaly, N.; Farokhzad, O. C., Cancer nanotechnology: The impact of passive and active targeting in the era of modern cancer biology. *Advanced Drug Delivery Reviews* 2014, 66, 2–25.
36. Rein, M. J.; Renouf, M.; Cruz-Hernandez, C.; Actis-Goretta, L.; Thakkar, S. K.; da Silva Pinto, M., Bioavailability of bioactive food compounds: A challenging journey to bioefficacy. *British Journal of Clinical Pharmacology* 2013, 75 (3), 588–602.
37. Pechanova, O.; Dayar, E.; Cebova, M., Therapeutic potential of polyphenols-loaded polymeric nanoparticles in cardiovascular system. *Molecules* 2020, 25 (15), 3322.
38. Izadpanah, A.; Gallo, R. L., Antimicrobial peptides. *Journal of the American Academy of Dermatology* 2005, 52 (3), 381–390.
39. Shai, Y., Mechanism of the binding, insertion and destabilization of phospholipid bilayer membranes by α-helical antimicrobial and cell non-selective membrane-lytic peptides. *Biochimica et Biophysica Acta (BBA)-Biomembranes* 1999, *1462* (1–2), 55–70.
40. Yang, L.; Harroun, T. A.; Weiss, T. M.; Ding, L.; Huang, H. W., Barrel-stave model or toroidal model? A case study on melittin pores. *Biophysical Journal* 2001, 81 (3), 1475–1485.
41. Wang, S.; Zeng, X.; Yang, Q.; Qiao, S., Antimicrobial peptides as potential alternatives to antibiotics in food animal industry. *International Journal of Molecular Sciences* 2016, 17 (5), 603.
42. Narayana, J. L.; Chen, J.-Y., Antimicrobial peptides: Possible anti-infective agents. *Peptides* 2015, 72, 88–94.
43. Sharma, A.; Gaur, A.; Kumar, V.; Sharma, N.; Patil, S. A.; Verma, R. K.; Singh, A. K., Antimicrobial activity of synthetic antimicrobial peptides loaded in poly-Ɛ-caprolactone nanoparticles against mycobacteria and their functional synergy with rifampicin. *International Journal of Pharmaceutics* 2021, 608, 121097.
44. Moghaddam, M. M.; Aghamollaei, H.; Kooshki, H.; Barjini, K. A.; Mirnejad, R.; Choopani, A., The development of antimicrobial peptides as an approach to prevention of antibiotic resistance. *Reviews and Research in Medical Microbiology* 2015, 26 (3), 98–110.
45. Oddo, A.; Hansen, P. R., Hemolytic activity of antimicrobial peptides. *Antimicrobial Peptides: Methods and Protocols* 2017, 1548, 427–435.
46. (a) Gómez-Sequeda, N.; Ruiz, J.; Ortiz, C.; Urquiza, M.; Torres, R., Potent and specific antibacterial activity against *Escherichia coli* O157:H7 and Methicillin Resistant Staphylococcus aureus (MRSA) of G17 and G19 peptides encapsulated into Poly-Lactic-Co-Glycolic Acid (PLGA) nanoparticles. *Antibiotics* 2020, *9* (7), 384; (b) Hemeg, H. A., Nanomaterials for alternative antibacterial therapy. *International Journal of Nanomedicine* 2017, 12, 8211–8225.
47. Gupta, A.; Bahal, R.; Gupta, M.; Glazer, P. M.; Saltzman, W. M., Nanotechnology for delivery of peptide nucleic acids (PNAs). *Journal of Controlled Release* 2016, 240, 302–311.
48. Bhatia, T.; Gupta, G. D.; Kurmi, B. D.; Singh, D., Role of solid lipid nanoparticles for the delivery of lipophilic drugs and herbal medicines in the treatment of pulmonary hypertension. *Pharmaceutical Nanotechnology* 2022, *10* (5), 342–353.

49. Delfi, M.; Sartorius, R.; Ashrafizadeh, M.; Sharifi, E.; Zhang, Y.; De Berardinis, P.; Zarrabi, A.; Varma, R. S.; Tay, F. R.; Smith, B. R., Self-assembled peptide and protein nanostructures for anti-cancer therapy: Targeted delivery, stimuli-responsive devices and immunotherapy. *Nano Today* 2021, *38*, 101119.
50. Zhao, Z.; Ukidve, A.; Kim, J.; Mitragotri, S., Targeting strategies for tissue-specific drug delivery. *Cell* 2020, *181* (1), 151–167.
51. Ruoslahti, E., Peptides as targeting elements and tissue penetration devices for nanoparticles. *Advanced Materials* 2012, 24 (28), 3747–3756.
52. Vasir, J. K.; Reddy, M. K.; Labhasetwar, V. D., Nanosystems in drug targeting: Opportunities and challenges. *Current Nanoscience* 2005, 1 (1), 47–64.
53. Mills, J. K.; Needham, D., Targeted drug delivery. *Expert Opinion on Therapeutic Patents* 1999, 9 (11), 1499–1513.
54. Garnett, M. C., Targeted drug conjugates: Principles and progress. *Advanced Drug Delivery Reviews* 2001, 53 (2), 171–216.
55. Petros, R. A.; DeSimone, J. M., Strategies in the design of nanoparticles for therapeutic applications. *Nature Reviews Drug Discovery* 2010, 9 (8), 615–627.
56. Martin, C.; Oyen, E.; Van Wanseele, Y.; Haddou, T. B.; Schmidhammer, H.; Andrade, J.; Waddington, L.; Van Eeckhaut, A.; Van Mele, B.; Gardiner, J., Injectable peptide-based hydrogel formulations for the extended in vivo release of opioids. *Materials Today Chemistry* 2017, 3, 49–59.
57. Jonker, A. M.; Löwik, D. W. P. M.; van Hest, J. C. M., Peptide- and protein-based hydrogels. *Chemistry of Materials* 2012, 24 (5), 759–773.
58. Bertilla, X. J.; Rupachandra, S., Insights into current directions of protein and peptide-based hydrogel drug delivery systems for inflammation. *Polymer Bulletin* 2022, 80, 9409–9436.
59. Miura, Y.; Takenaka, T.; Toh, K.; Wu, S.; Nishihara, H.; Kano, M. R.; Ino, Y.; Nomoto, T.; Matsumoto, Y.; Koyama, H., Cyclic RGD-linked polymeric micelles for targeted delivery of platinum anticancer drugs to glioblastoma through the blood–brain tumor barrier. *ACS Nano* 2013, 7 (10), 8583–8592.
60. Alipour, M.; Baneshi, M.; Hosseinkhani, S.; Mahmoudi, R.; Jabari Arabzadeh, A.; Akrami, M.; Mehrzad, J.; Bardania, H., Recent progress in biomedical applications of RGD-based ligand: From precise cancer theranostics to biomaterial engineering: A systematic review. *Journal of Biomedical Materials Research Part A* 2020, 108 (4), 839–850.
61. Pirooznia, N.; Abdi, K.; Beiki, D.; Emami, F.; Arab, S. S.; Sabzevari, O.; Pakdin-Parizi, Z.; Geramifar, P., Radiosynthesis, biological evaluation, and preclinical study of a 68 Ga-labeled cyclic RGD peptide as an early diagnostic agent for overexpressed α v β 3 integrin receptors in non-small-cell lung cancer. *Contrast Media & Molecular Imaging* 2020, 1, 8421657. 62. Bolhassani, A., Potential efficacy of cell-penetrating peptides for nucleic acid and drug delivery in cancer. *Biochimica et Biophysica Acta (BBA)-Reviews on Cancer* 2011, *1816* (2), 232–246.
63. Nasrollahi, S. A.; Taghibiglou, C.; Azizi, E.; Farboud, E. S., Cell-penetrating peptides as a novel transdermal drug delivery system. *Chemical Biology & Drug Design* 2012, 80 (5), 639–646.
64. Skotland, T.; Iversen, T. G.; Torgersen, M. L.; Sandvig, K., Cell-penetrating peptides: Possibilities and challenges for drug delivery in vitro and in vivo. *Molecules* 2015, *20* (7), 13313–13323.
65. Doering, T.; Holleran, W. M.; Potratz, A.; Vielhaber, G.; Elias, P. M.; Suzuki, K.; Sandhoff, K., Sphingolipid activator proteins are required for epidermal permeability barrier formation. *The Journal of Biological Chemistry* 1999, 274 (16), 11038–45.

66. Fonseca, S. B.; Pereira, M. P.; Kelley, S. O., Recent advances in the use of cell-penetrating peptides for medical and biological applications. *Advanced Drug Delivery Reviews* 2009, 61 (11), 953–964.
67. Vives, E.; Brodin, P.; Lebleu, B., A truncated HIV-1 Tat protein basic domain rapidly translocates through the plasma membrane and accumulates in the cell nucleus. *Journal of Biological Chemistry* 1997, 272 (25), 16010–16017.
68. Joliot, A.; Prochiantz, A., Transduction peptides: From technology to physiology. *Nature Cell Biology* 2004, 6 (3), 189–196.
69. Urandur, S.; Sullivan, M. O., Peptide-based vectors: A biomolecular engineering strategy for gene delivery. *Annual Review of Chemical and Biomolecular Engineering* 2023, 14, 243–264.
70. Morris, M. C.; Deshayes, S.; Heitz, F.; Divita, G., Cell-penetrating peptides: From molecular mechanisms to therapeutics. *Biology of the Cell* 2008, 100 (4), 201–217.
71. Derossi, D.; Joliot, A. H.; Chassaing, G.; Prochiantz, A., The third helix of the Antennapedia homeodomain translocates through biological membranes. *Journal of Biological Chemistry* 1994, 269 (14), 10444–10450.
72. Fawell, S.; Seery, J.; Daikh, Y.; Moore, C.; Chen, L. L.; Pepinsky, B.; Barsoum, J., Tat-mediated delivery of heterologous proteins into cells. *Proceedings of the National Academy of Sciences* 1994, 91 (2), 664–668.
73. Wender, P. A.; Mitchell, D. J.; Pattabiraman, K.; Pelkey, E. T.; Steinman, L.; Rothbard, J. B., The design, synthesis, and evaluation of molecules that enable or enhance cellular uptake: Peptoid molecular transporters. *Proceedings of the National Academy of Sciences* 2000, 97 (24), 13003–13008.
74. Pooga, M.; Hällbrink, M.; Zorko, M.; Langel, Ü., Cell penetration by transportan. *The FASEB Journal* 1998, 12 (1), 67–77.
75. Madani, F.; Lindberg, S.; Langel, Ü.; Futaki, S.; Gräslund, A., Mechanisms of cellular uptake of cell-penetrating peptides. *Journal of Biophysics* 2011, 1, 414729..
76. Qian, Y.; Billeter, M.; Otting, G.; Müller, M.; Gehring, W.; Wüthrich, K., The structure of the Antennapedia homeodomain determined by NMR spectroscopy in solution: Comparison with prokaryotic repressors. *Cell* 1989, *59* (3), 573–580.
77. Wang, F.; Wang, Y.; Zhang, X.; Zhang, W.; Guo, S.; Jin, F., Recent progress of cell-penetrating peptides as new carriers for intracellular cargo delivery. *Journal of Controlled Release* 2014, 174, 126–136.
78. Farkhani, S. M.; Valizadeh, A.; Karami, H.; Mohammadi, S.; Sohrabi, N.; Badrzadeh, F., Cell penetrating peptides: Efficient vectors for delivery of nanoparticles, nanocarriers, therapeutic and diagnostic molecules. *Peptides* 2014, 57, 78–94.
79. Laracuente, M.-L.; Marina, H. Y.; McHugh, K. J., Zero-order drug delivery: State of the art and future prospects. *Journal of Controlled Release* 2020, 327, 834–856.
80. Lundberg, P.; El-Andaloussi, S.; Sütlü, T.; Johansson, H.; Langel, Ü., Delivery of short interfering RNA using endosomolytic cell-penetrating peptides. *The FASEB Journal* 2007, 21 (11), 2664–2671.
81. Juliano, R. L.; Alam, R.; Dixit, V.; Kang, H. M., Cell-targeting and cell-penetrating peptides for delivery of therapeutic and imaging agents. *Wiley Interdisciplinary Reviews: Nanomedicine and Nanobiotechnology* 2009, 1 (3), 324–335.
82. Medintz, I. L.; Pons, T.; Delehanty, J. B.; Susumu, K.; Brunel, F. M.; Dawson, P. E.; Mattoussi, H., Intracellular delivery of quantum dot–protein cargos mediated by cell penetrating peptides. *Bioconjugate Chemistry* 2008, *19* (9), 1785–1795.
83. Shin, M. C.; Zhang, J.; Min, K. A.; Lee, K.; Byun, Y.; David, A. E.; He, H.; Yang, V. C., Cell-penetrating peptides: Achievements and challenges in application for cancer treatment. *Journal of Biomedical Materials Research Part A: An Official Journal*

84. Iqbal, J.; Anwar, F.; Afridi, S., Targeted drug delivery systems and their therapeutic applications in cancer and immune pathological conditions. *Infectious Disorders-Drug Targets (Formerly Current Drug Targets-Infectious Disorders)* 2017, *17* (3), 149–159.
85. Yang, R.; Wei, T.; Goldberg, H.; Wang, W.; Cullion, K.; Kohane, D. S., Getting drugs across biological barriers. *Advanced Materials* 2017, *29* (37), 1606596.
86. Bazak, R.; Houri, M.; El Achy, S.; Hussein, W.; Refaat, T., Passive targeting of nanoparticles to cancer: A comprehensive review of the literature. *Molecular and Clinical Oncology* 2014, 2 (6), 904–908.
87. Goyal, R.; Ramakrishnan, V., Chapter 2- peptide-based drug delivery systems. In *Characterization and biology of nanomaterials for drug delivery*, Mohapatra, S. S.; Ranjan, S.; Dasgupta, N.; Mishra, R. K.; Thomas, S., Eds. Elsevier: 2019; pp. 25–45.
88. Singh, A. P.; Biswas, A.; Shukla, A.; Maiti, P., Targeted therapy in chronic diseases using nanomaterial-based drug delivery vehicles. *Signal Transduction and Targeted Therapy* 2019, *4* (1), 33.
89. Naqvi, S.; Panghal, A.; Flora, S., Nanotechnology: A promising approach for delivery of neuroprotective drugs. *Frontiers in Neuroscience* 2020, *14*, 494.
90. Saranya, S.; Laksiri, W., The Role of Nanotechnology in Understanding the Pathophysiology of Traumatic Brain Injury, *Central Nervous System Agents in Medicinal Chemistry* 2025, 25 (1), e250424229330. DOI: 10.2174/0118715249291 999240418112531
91. Vyas, S. P.; Singh, A.; Sihorkar, V., Ligand-receptor-mediated drug delivery: An emerging paradigm in cellular drug targeting. *Critical Reviews™ in Therapeutic Drug Carrier Systems* 2001, *18* (1), 76.
92. Hu, Q.; Katti, P. S.; Gu, Z., Enzyme-responsive nanomaterials for controlled drug delivery. *Nanoscale* 2014, *6* (21), 12273–12286.
93. Bareford, L. M.; Swaan, P. W., Endocytic mechanisms for targeted drug delivery. *Advanced Drug Delivery Reviews* 2007, 59 (8), 748–758.
94. Aqil, F.; Munagala, R.; Jeyabalan, J.; Vadhanam, M. V., Bioavailability of phytochemicals and its enhancement by drug delivery systems. *Cancer Letters* 2013, *334* (1), 133–141.
95. Maeda, H., The enhanced permeability and retention (EPR) effect in tumor vascularture: The key role of tumor-selective macromolecular drug targeting. *Advances in Enzyme Regulation* 2001, *41*, 1898–1207.
96. Cho, K.; Wang, X.; Nie, S.; Chen, Z. G.; Shin, D. M., Therapeutic nanoparticles for drug delivery in cancer. *Clinical Cancer Research: An Official Journal of the American Association for Cancer Research* 2008, *14* (5), 1310–1316.
97. Roma, P.; Amandeep, G.; Pankaj, B., Chronic inflammation. *StatPearls* https://www.ncbi.nlm.nih.gov/books/NBK493173/.
98. Mao, J.; Ran, D.; Xie, C.; Shen, Q.; Wang, S.; Lu, W., EGFR/EGFRvIII dual-targeting peptide-mediated drug delivery for enhanced glioma therapy. *ACS Applied Materials & Interfaces* 2017, *9* (29), 24462–24475.
99. Jafari, B.; Pourseif, M. M.; Barar, J.; Rafi, M. A.; Omidi, Y., Peptide-mediated drug delivery across the blood-brain barrier for targeting brain tumors. *Expert Opinion on Drug Delivery* 2019, 16 (6), 583–605.

100. Jia, R.; Teng, L.; Gao, L.; Su, T.; Fu, L.; Qiu, Z.; Bi, Y., Advances in multiple stimuli-responsive drug-delivery systems for cancer therapy. *International Journal of Nanomedicine* 2021, 16, 1525–1551.
101. Darvin, P.; Chandrasekharan, A.; Santhosh Kumar, T. R., Chapter 1- Introduction to smart drug delivery systems. In *Biomimetic nanoengineered materials for advanced drug delivery*, Unnithan, A. R.; Sasikala, A. R. K.; Park, C. H.; Kim, C. S., Eds. Elsevier: 2019; pp. 1–9.
102. Li, F.; Qin, Y.; Lee, J.; Liao, H.; Wang, N.; Davis, T. P.; Qiao, R.; Ling, D., Stimuli-responsive nano-assemblies for remotely controlled drug delivery. *Journal of Controlled Release* 2020, 322, 566–592.
103. Ganta, S.; Devalapally, H.; Shahiwala, A.; Amiji, M., A review of stimuli-responsive nanocarriers for drug and gene delivery. *Journal of Controlled Release* 2008, 126 (3), 187–204.
104. Li, Y.; Zhang, C.; Li, G.; Deng, G.; Zhang, H.; Sun, Y.; An, F., Protease-triggered bioresponsive drug delivery for the targeted theranostics of malignancy. *Acta Pharmaceutica Sinica B* 2021, 11 (8), 2220–2242.
105. Bisoyi, H. K.; Li, Q., Liquid crystals: Versatile self-organized smart soft materials. *Chemical Reviews* 2022, 122 (5), 4887–4926.
106. Yu, K.; Mei, Y.; Hadjesfandiari, N.; Kizhakkedathu, J. N., Engineering biomaterials surfaces to modulate the host response. *Colloids and Surfaces B: Biointerfaces* 2014, 124, 69–79.
107. Gondi, C. S.; Rao, J. S., Cathepsin B as a cancer target. *Expert Opinion on Therapeutic Targets* 2013, 17 (3), 281–291.
108. Zhang, C.; Pan, D.; Li, J.; Hu, J.; Bains, A.; Guys, N.; Zhu, H.; Li, X.; Luo, K.; Gong, Q.; Gu, Z., Enzyme-responsive peptide dendrimer-gemcitabine conjugate as a controlled-release drug delivery vehicle with enhanced antitumor efficacy. *Acta Biomaterialia* 2017, 55, 153–162.
109. Berillo, D.; Yeskendir, A.; Zharkinbekov, Z.; Raziyeva, K.; Saparov, A., Peptide-based drug delivery systems. *Medicina* 2021, 57 (11), 1209.
110. Gaspar, D.; Veiga, A. S.; Castanho, M. A., From antimicrobial to anticancer peptides. A review. *Frontiers in Microbiology* 2013, 4, 294.
111. Norouzi, P.; Mirmohammadi, M.; Tehrani, M. H. H., Anticancer peptides mechanisms, simple and complex. *Chemico-Biological Interactions* 2022, 368, 110194, ISSN 0009-2797.
112. Xie, M.; Liu, D.; Yang, Y., Anti-cancer peptides: Classification, mechanism of action, reconstruction and modification. *Open Biology* 2020, 10 (7), 200004.
113. Tian, G.; Sobotka-Briner, C. D.; Zysk, J.; Liu, X.; Birr, C.; Sylvester, M. A.; Edwards, P. D.; Scott, C. D.; Greenberg, B. D., Linear non-competitive inhibition of solubilized human γ-secretase by pepstatin A methylester, L685458, sulfonamides, and benzodiazepines. *Journal of Biological Chemistry* 2002, 277 (35), 31499–31505.
114. Patocka, J.; Nepovimova, E.; Klimova, B.; Wu, Q.; Kuca, K., Antimicrobial peptides: Amphibian host defense peptides. *Current Medicinal Chemistry* 2019, 26 (32), 5924–5946.
115. Bojarska, J., Advances in research of short peptides. *Molecules* 2022, 27 (8), 2446.
116. Diamond, G.; Beckloff, N.; Weinberg, A.; Kisich, K. O., The roles of antimicrobial peptides in innate host defense. *Current Pharmaceutical Design* 2009, 15 (21), 2377–2392.
117. Dürr, U. H.; Sudheendra, U.; Ramamoorthy, A., LL-37, the only human member of the cathelicidin family of antimicrobial peptides. *Biochimica et Biophysica Acta (BBA)-Biomembranes* 2006, 1758 (9), 1408–1425.

118. Santos, J. C.; Sousa, R. C.; Otoni, C. G.; Moraes, A. R.; Souza, V. G.; Medeiros, E. A.; Espitia, P. J.; Pires, A. C.; Coimbra, J. S.; Soares, N. F., Nisin and other antimicrobial peptides: Production, mechanisms of action, and application in active food packaging. *Innovative Food Science & Emerging Technologies* 2018, 48, 179–194.
119. Tornesello, A. L.; Borrelli, A.; Buonaguro, L.; Buonaguro, F. M.; Tornesello, M. L., Antimicrobial peptides as anticancer agents: Functional properties and biological activities. *Molecules* 2020, *25* (12), 2850.
120. Kluskens, L. D.; Nelemans, S. A.; Rink, R.; Vries, L. D.; Meter-Arkema, A.; Wang, Y.; Walther, T.; Kuipers, A.; Moll, G. N.; Haas, M., Angiotensin-(1–7) with Thioether Bridge: An angiotensin-converting enzyme-resistant, potent angiotensin-(1–7) analog. *Journal of Pharmacology and Experimental Therapeutics* 2009, 328 (3), 849–854.
121. Zhang, L.; Huang, Y.; Lindstrom, A. R.; Lin, T. Y.; Lam, K. S.; Li, Y., Peptide-based materials for cancer immunotherapy. *Theranostics* 2019, *9* (25), 7807–7825.
122. Barua, S.; Mitragotri, S., Challenges associated with penetration of nanoparticles across cell and tissue barriers: A review of current status and future prospects. *Nano Today* 2014, 9 (2), 223–243.
123. Jain, K. K., Personalised medicine for cancer: From drug development into clinical practice. *Expert Opinion on Pharmacotherapy* 2005, 6 (9), 1463–1476.
124. Xiao, Y.-F.; Jie, M.-M.; Li, B.-S.; Hu, C.-J.; Xie, R.; Tang, B.; Yang, S.-M., Peptide-based treatment: A promising cancer therapy. *Journal of Immunology Research* 2015, *2015*, 761820.
125. Kim, E.-S.; Ahn, E. H.; Dvir, T.; Kim, D.-H., Emerging nanotechnology approaches in tissue engineering and regenerative medicine. *International Journal of Nanomedicine* 2014, 9 (supl), 1–5.

5 Applications of peptide-conjugated nanomaterials

5.1 GENERAL APPLICATIONS OF PEPTIDE-CONJUGATED NANOMATERIALS

As discussed in Chapter 4, we understand there are many forms of peptide-conjugated nanomaterials. In this chapter, we will discuss the potential applications in a wide range of fields of peptide-conjugated nanomaterials, such as medicine, biotechnology, and materials science. Here are some of the most promising applications (Figure 5.1). Overall, the applications of peptide-conjugated nanomaterials are diverse and promising, with the potential to revolutionize various fields of science and medicine as described in Table 5.1.

5.2 INTRODUCTION TO PEPTIDE-BASED SENSORS AND BIOSENSORS

Peptide-based sensors and biosensors are emerging technologies that offer significant advantages over traditional sensing methods. These sensing devices are intended to detect a broad spectrum of biomolecules with high sensitivity and specificity, including proteins, DNA, and tiny molecules.[9] Peptide-based sensors

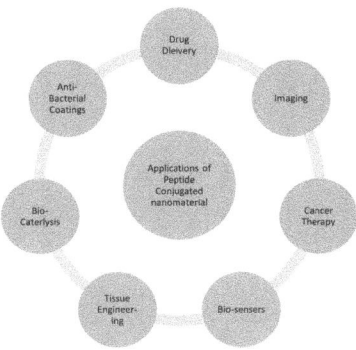

FIGURE 5.1 General application of peptide-conjugated nanomaterials.

TABLE 5.1
Overview of the applications of peptide-conjugated nanomaterials

Application	Comment	Examples	Ref
Drug delivery	Peptides conjugated with nanoparticles where drugs are capable of being delivered to specific cells or tissues in the body using this method, increasing their effectiveness while reducing side effects.	To promote the nuclear import of Chimeric Antigen Receptor (CAR)-encoding DNA, poly(β-amino ester) (PBAE)-based nanoparticles were used to carry DNA cargo into the nucleus of T cells and were further functionalized with peptides comprising microtubule-associated sequences and nuclear localization signals.	1
Imaging	Nanoparticles loaded with peptides can be utilized as contrast agents in medical imaging, such as MRI and computed tomography (CT) scans.	The deposition of Aβ peptides in the brain is one of the pathological characteristics of Alzheimer's disease, a neurodegenerative disease that causes progressive and irreversible loss of mental abilities.	2,3
Cancer therapy	Peptide-conjugated nanoparticles can be used to target cancer cells, delivering drugs or other therapies directly to the tumor site.	Employing a water-soluble, amine-to-sulfhydryl crosslinker, checkpoint inhibitors were linked to a peptide generated from placental growth factor 2 (PLGF2), which has an extraordinarily high affinity for numerous matrix proteins.	4
Biosensors	Peptides can be conjugated with nanomaterials to create highly sensitive biosensors for detecting various biomolecules, including proteins and DNA.	Numerous sensitive fluorophores may respond quickly to environmental changes and stimulation, which reflect a shift in spectrum properties. Environmentally sensitive fluorophores have become widely employed as signal markers to conjugate to peptides in order to develop peptide-based molecular sensors.	5
Tissue engineering	Peptide-conjugated nanomaterials can be used to create scaffolds that support the growth of new tissue, making them useful in tissue engineering applications.	A biomimetic Zein polydopamine-based nanofiber substrate was created to deliver bone morphogenic protein-2 (BMP-2) peptide-attributed titanium dioxide nanoparticles over an extended period with the intent to study their osteogenic differentiation potential.	6
Biocatalysis	Peptide-nanomaterial conjugates can be used as highly efficient biocatalysts for various chemical reactions.	Surface-functionalized single-enzyme metal-organic frameworks (MOF) particles are surface-functionalized with complementary peptides, whereby the self-assembled peptide coiled-coil structure induces MOF particle super-assembly, providing different enzyme-containing MOF particles together to trigger two- or three-enzyme cascade reactions.	7
Antibacterial coatings	Peptide-conjugated nanomaterials can be used to create coatings for medical devices or surfaces that are highly effective at preventing bacterial growth and infection.	Polylactic acid (PLA)-coated and Low-Density Lipoprotein Receptor (LDLR) ligand peptide-functionalized mesoporous silica nanoparticles (MSNPs) are a delivery mechanism that can actively cross the BBB via receptor-mediated transcytosis and release antioxidant Respiratory syncytial virus (RSV) upon reactive oxygen species (ROS) stimulation to treat neurological diseases that arise from oxidative stress.	8

and biosensors are also highly selective, allowing for the revealing of specific biomolecules in complex biological samples, such as blood or urine.[10]

As peptides are short-chain sequences of amino acids, they are the fundamental units of proteins. Peptides are highly versatile and may be constructed for use with specific properties, such as binding to specific molecules or cells. Peptides can also be synthesized with various functional groups, allowing for the conjugation of peptides with various materials, including nanoparticles, polymers, and surfaces. This is one main reason why peptides are effective as sensing elements in biosensors have gained due to their distinctive characteristics; they have received a lot of attention over the past few years. Peptides can be further designed to recognize specific targets with high affinity and selectivity, adapted as ideal candidates for use in biosensors. In addition, peptides are stable and easily synthesized and can be modified to improve their performance.

Biosensors are tools that combine physical transducers with biological recognition components to transform biological data into observable signals for quantitative or semiquantitative analysis. Most people consider sensitivity, selectivity, and stability to be the most important.[11] Biosensors were described as "Analytical devices incorporating a biological material either associated with or integrated within, a physiochemical transducer or transducing microsystem" during the 10th World Congress on the Biosensors, which was held in Shanghai, China, in 2008. The transducer could be magnetic, micromechanical, electrochemical, piezoelectric, or optical.[12] A typical biosensor is made up of three fundamental components: (1) a biological recognition unit that contacts with a specific target, (2) a transducer that converts a solution or surface property into a recordable signal, and (3) an electronic system that records and analyzes this signal and translates it into an analog/digital display (Figures 5.2 and 5.3). Significant advancements in developing new biosensors that can offer very sensitive, accurate, and painless diagnostics have been noted over the past few years. Although biosensors were initially utilized mostly in the healthcare and medical industries, with important equipment used for uses such as diabetes monitoring, pregnancy detection, and cardiac monitoring, they are now used for a wide range of applications; they have recently spread to a variety of industries, including agriculture, environmental monitoring, security, and biodefense.[13,14]

However, peptide-based biosensors typically consist of two components: a peptide that acts as the recognition element and a transducer that turns the binding process into a signal. The transducer can be an optical, electrochemical, or mechanical sensor, depending on the type of signal to be measured.[15]

Optical sensors are the most commonly used transducers in peptide-based biosensors.[16] Optical sensors rely on the changes in light intensity, wavelength, or polarization that occurs when a biomolecule binds to the peptide. Fluorescence, surface plasmon resonance (SPR), and colorimetric assays are examples of optical sensors used in peptide-based biosensors.[17] When the analyte is delivered close to the sensing device, these sensors exhibit their unique optical resonance signature, such as a modification in refractive index. The optical resonance of the sensor shifts in frequency when the refractive index changes.[18]

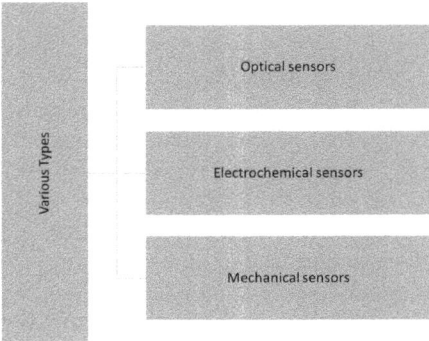

FIGURE 5.2 Types of biosensors.

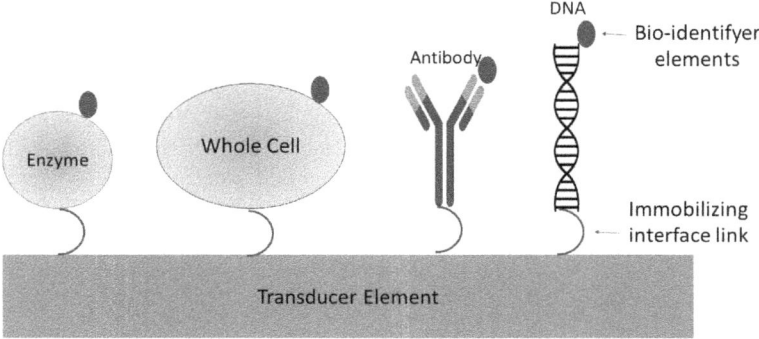

FIGURE 5.3 The different forms of biosensors and the interaction between the target bio identifier element.

Electrochemical sensors are also commonly used in peptide-based biosensors. Electrochemical sensors rely on the changes in current or voltage that occurs when a biomolecule binds to the peptide. Electrochemical sensors are highly sensitive and selective, making them ideal for the finding of biomolecules in complex samples.[19] The exact mechanisms behind these responses are frequently not known. The presence of an analyte molecule causes a measurable alteration in the current flow. The potential difference is observed in the case of a field-effect biosensor; this is manifested as a change in conductance elsewhere in the apparatus, such as across a film of an underlying semiconductor.[20,21]

On the other hand, mechanical sensors are the newest type of transducer used in peptide-based biosensors. These sensors rely on the alterations in the mechanical properties of the peptide or the substrate when a biomolecule binds to the peptide. These sensors are highly sensitive and can be used to detect very small amounts of biomolecules.[22] The chemical reaction of graphene with several typical silk fibroin peptide structures extracted from different domains of silk fibroin, including pure amorphous (P1), pure crystalline (P2), an N-terminal segment (P3), and a combined amorphous and crystalline segment (P4), alongside the objective of revealing structural modifications, while graphene can have intriguing influences on the structures formed by the peptides with sequences representing different domains of silk fibroin.[23]

Peptide-based biosensors have numerous possibilities for use, including medical diagnostics, environmental monitoring, and food safety. In medical diagnostics, peptide-based biosensors can be used for the early detection of diseases, such as cancer, cardiovascular diseases, and infectious diseases.[24] Peptide-based biosensors can also be used for the monitoring of therapeutic drugs and their metabolites in patients. When creating therapeutic drug monitoring (TDM) sensing components, short peptides provide a practical substitute for aptamers since they are simple to synthesize in large quantities, inexpensive, and biostable.[25]

While, in environmental monitoring, peptide-based biosensors can be used for the detection of heavy metals, herbicides, and poisons that have been detected in water and soil samples, they can also be applied for the observation of pathogens in food and water.[26] It is traditionally performed using either naturally occurring or manufactured protein molecules and involves metal ion sensing. For instance, metallothionein, a metal-binding protein that comes from mammals, has been combined into an optical biosensor for the nondiscriminatory detection of cadmium, zinc, or nickel.[27]

The development of peptide-based biosensors is a rapidly growing field of research, with new peptide sequences and sensor designs being developed every year. The combination of peptides with various transducers is leading to the development of biosensors with high sensitivity, specificity, and selectivity. Peptide-based biosensors have the potential to revolutionize the way we detect and monitor biomolecules, making them a powerful tool in many scientific and medical applications.

5.2.1 Peptide-based biosensors for disease diagnosis, environmental monitoring, and food quality control

Peptide-based biosensors have developed as a powerful tool for the detection and monitoring of biomolecules in a wide range of fields, including disease diagnosis, environmental monitoring, and food quality control. The unique properties of peptides, such as high specificity and selectivity, make them ideal applicants for use in biosensors. In this section, we will discuss the applications of peptide-based biosensors in disease diagnosis, environmental monitoring, and food quality control.

5.2.1.1 Disease diagnosis

Peptide-based biosensors have shown great promise in the early detection of diseases, such as cancer, cardiovascular diseases, and infectious diseases. They are highly sensitive and can detect very small amounts of biomolecules, allowing for the observations of diseases at an early stage when treatment is most effective.[28]

One example of a peptide-based biosensor for disease diagnosis is the detection of prostate-specific antigen (PSA) in blood samples.[29] PSA is a biomarker for prostate cancer (PCa), and the early detection of PSA can lead to early diagnosis and treatment. A peptide sequence that binds specifically to PSA was rented into a gold nanoparticle, and the resulting biosensor was able to detect PSA at a concentration as low as 2 ng/mL. This biosensor has an opportunity to assist in the early detection of diseases such as PCa, leading to better patient outcomes.[30]

Another example of a peptide-based biosensor for disease diagnosis is the detection of troponin, a biomarker for cardiovascular diseases.[28] Troponin is released into the bloodstream after a heart attack, and the early prognostic of troponin can lead to early diagnosis and treatment. A peptide sequence that binds specifically to troponin was conjugated to an SPR sensor, and the resulting biosensor was used to detect troponin at a concentration as low as 1 ng/mL. This biosensor has the potential to be used in the early discovery of cardiovascular diseases, leading to better patient outcomes.[31]

5.2.1.2 Environmental monitoring

Peptide-based biosensors can also be used for the detection of pollutants, such as heavy metals, pesticides, and toxins, in water and soil samples. They are highly selective and can detect specific pollutants in complex environmental samples.[32] The development of portable sensors that can monitor wastewater on-site is made possible by the miniaturization of biosensors. Various forms of biosensors are divided into (1) electrochemical, (2) optical, (3) piezoelectric, and (4) thermal biosensors based on their transducing mechanisms. This is done in consideration of the wide range of biorecognition methods (including immunochemical, enzymatic, nonenzymatic receptor, molecularly imprinted polymer (MIP), whole cell, and DNA elements).[33]

One example of a peptide-based biosensor for environmental monitoring is the discovery of mercury in water samples. Mercury is a toxic heavy metal that can contaminate water sources and pose a threat to human health.[34] A peptide sequence that binds specifically to mercury was conjugated to a carbon nanotube-based sensor, and the resulting biosensor was capable of distinguishing mercury at a concentration as low as 10 ng/L. This biosensor has the potential to be used in the monitoring of mercury contamination in water sources, leading to better environmental management.[35]

Another example of a peptide-based biosensor for environmental monitoring is the detection of glyphosate, a widely used herbicide, in soil samples. Glyphosate can have negative impacts on soil quality and the environment. A peptide sequence that binds specifically to glyphosate was conjugated to a fluorescence-based sensor, and the resulting biosensor was able to detect glyphosate at a concentration as low as 0.1 µM. This biosensor has the potential to be used in the monitoring of glyphosate contamination in soil, leading to better environmental management.[36]

5.2.13 Food quality control

Peptide-based biosensors are accomplished for pathogen detection and toxins in food samples, improving food safety and quality control. Peptide-based biosensors are highly selective and can detect specific pathogens and toxins in complex food samples,[37] such as the usage of Aantimicrobial peptides (AMPs) as sensors. When lipid bilayer disruption processes take place, AMP-based sensors inject the peptide into the cytoplasmic membrane after being electrostatically immobilized on the substrates. As a result, the peptides' permeability and capacity for transporting the cellular membrane may be hampered. It is challenging to distinguish the similarities and differences in the effects of soluble and immobilized AMPs due to the scarcity of experimental data on these compounds. More attention has been paid to AMPs' high affinity as recognition components for bacterial surfaces in the development of sensors than to their antibacterial action.[37,38]

One example of a peptide-based biosensor for food quality control is the detection of *Salmonella*, a common pathogen in poultry and eggs. *Salmonella* contamination in food can lead to foodborne illness and endanger the public's health. A peptide sequence that binds specifically to *Salmonella* was capable of spotting was conjugated to a magnetic bead-based sensor, and the resulting biosensor was able to detect *Salmonella* at a concentration as low as 1 cfu/mL in chicken samples. This biosensor has the possibility of being employed in identifying the presence of a variety of *Salmonella* contamination in food products, leading to improved food safety and quality control.[39]

Another example of a peptide-based biosensor in food quality control is the detection of histamine, a toxin produced by bacteria in spoiled fish. Histamine contamination in food can cause food poisoning and pose a threat to human health. A peptide sequence that binds specifically to histamine was conjugated to an SPR sensor, and the resulting biosensor was able to detect histamine at a concentration as low as 0.3 µM in tuna samples. This biosensor has the possibility of being employed in identifying histamine contamination in seafood products, leading to improved food safety and quality control.[40]

Peptide-based biosensors are applied in various forms such as in disease diagnosis, environmental monitoring, and food quality control. Peptide-based biosensors are highly selective and sensitive, allowing for the detection of specific biomolecules in complex samples. The use of peptide-based biosensors has the potential to improve patient outcomes, environmental management, and food safety and quality control, making them a valuable tool in various fields. Additional study and development in this area may result in the advancement of even more advanced peptide-based biosensors with even greater sensitivity and specificity, improving our ability to detect and monitor biomolecules in a variety of applications.

5.3 INTRODUCTION TO PEPTIDE-BASED TISSUE ENGINEERING AND REGENERATIVE MEDICINE

Peptide-based tissue engineering and regenerative medicine is an emerging connection in field principles of biomaterials, cell biology, and engineering to create functional tissues and organs for the repair and replacement of damaged or diseased tissues.[41] Peptide amino acid sequences can be engineered to mimic the extracellular matrix (ECM), which is the natural scaffold that provides mechanical support and signaling cues for cells in tissues.[42] Peptide-based materials can be designed to promote cell adhesion, proliferation, differentiation, and tissue remodeling, making them attractive candidates for tissue engineering and regenerative medicine applications.[43]

The use of peptides in tissue engineering and regenerative medicine has several advantages over traditional approaches. Peptides can be synthesized with high purity and consistency, allowing for precise control over their properties and functions. Peptides are biocompatible and biodegradable, reducing the threat of immunogenicity and toxicity. Peptides can also be modified with functional groups, such as growth factors and cell adhesion molecules, to enhance their biological activity and specificity.

The production of new tissues is one of the most difficult obstacles in tissue engineering and regenerative medicine of functional vascularized tissues, which require the formation of blood vessels to provide oxygen and nutrients to the cells.[44] Peptide-based materials can be designed to promote the formation of new blood vessels, a process known as angiogenesis.[45] A new blood vessel will branch off an existing blood vessel as part of the physiological process known as angiogenesis, which denotes the remodeling of vascular tissue. It is closely linked to the migration and growth of endothelial cells (ECs). While EC turnover is very low and restricted to specific physiologic events in adults, it is particularly active during embryonic development.[46] Proangiogenic and antiangiogenic factors regulate angiogenesis in a healthy person, and the deviation from this equilibrium (angiogenic switch) caused by certain stimuli, such as hypoxia, is linked to several human disorders (pathologic angiogenesis). Proliferating retinopathy, cancer, rheumatoid arthritis (RA), and psoriasis are all diseases that are characterized by the presence of proangiogenic factors (excessive angiogenesis), whereas coronary disorders, ischemia, and a decreased ability to regenerate tissue are all caused by a lack of angiogenesis.[47] Peptides can stimulate angiogenesis by binding to and activating specific receptors on ECs, which are the cells that line the inside of blood vessels. There have been reports of many peptides modulating vascular endothelial growth factor (VEGF)-dependent angiogenesis. They either bind to the ligand or the extracellular portion of the VEGF receptors. Only a small percentage of them displayed agonistic behavior; the majority exhibited antagonistic conduct. To produce peptides that disrupt the binding of the VEGF receptors, phage display libraries have been extensively used in screening.[48]

Peptide-based materials can also be designed to mimic the physical and chemical cues of the ECM that are important for angiogenesis, such as stiffness, topography, and chemical gradients.[49] Peptide-based materials have been utilized in a range of tissue engineering applications and regenerative medicine applications, including bone, cartilage, muscle, nerve, and skin tissue engineering.[50] For example, peptide-based hydrogels have been used to promote the regeneration of bone tissue by providing a three-dimensional (3D) scaffold for the attachment and proliferation of bone-forming cells, such as osteoblasts.[51] Cross-linked hydrophilic chain networks make up hydrogels, which are polymeric networks. Because of its great affinity for water, it has physical characteristics that allow it to absorb huge amounts of water or biological fluids while virtually staying insoluble. Since injectable hydrogels can replicate the ECM architecture and are typically biocompatible, biodegradable, and convenient to use in clinical settings, they have been developed as promising biomaterials for tissue engineering applications. As cellular therapies advance, there is a growing need to create injectable hydrogels that can carry cells. This will eliminate the need for open surgery and enable the use of minimally invasive methods to apply biomaterial and cells.[52] Peptide-based scaffolds are applied to promote the regeneration of cartilage tissue by providing a matrix that mimics the structure and properties of native cartilage. Peptide-based materials have also been used to promote the regeneration of nerve tissue by providing a scaffold that promotes the growth and guidance of nerve cells.[53]

In addition to tissue engineering, peptide-based materials have also been used in drug delivery and gene therapy applications. Peptides can be used as targeting ligands that bind to specific receptors on cells, enabling the delivery of therapeutic molecules to the desired site of action.[54] The targets can be found in the nucleus (DNA, antisense oligonucleotides, DNA intercalating agents like doxorubicin), cytoplasm (glucocorticoid receptors, proteins, and siRNA), mitochondria (antioxidants), or other subcellular regions of a cell. Furthermore, cytosolic administration is preferred for medications that are extensively effluxed from cells by efflux transporters such as P-glycoproteins (P-gp) and multidrug resistance proteins (MRPs). Recombinant proteins and plasmid DNA are two examples of macromolecular medications whose sites of action are typically the cytoplasm and nucleus, respectively. The ultimate goal of gene delivery can be realized only when the plasmid DNA can locate and combine with the nuclear or mitochondrial DNA. Additionally, as these medicinal substances are particularly vulnerable to enzymatic degradation, delivery mechanisms must be developed.[55] Hence, peptides can also be used as carriers for gene therapy vectors, such as plasmid DNA and viral vectors, to enhance their specificity and efficiency.[56]

Hence we understand that peptide-based tissue engineering and regenerative medicine is a promising field that has the potential to transform the medical management of many diseases and injuries. Peptides offer unique advantages in terms of biocompatibility, biodegradability, and functionality, making them attractive candidates for tissue engineering and regenerative medicine applications. The use of peptide-based materials provides the potential to enhance patient outcomes, reduce healthcare costs, and address critical medical needs.

5.3.1 PEPTIDE-BASED BIOMATERIAL SCAFFOLDS AND HYDROGELS FOR TISSUE ENGINEERING

Peptide-based biomaterial scaffolds and hydrogels have shown tremendous potential because of their capacity to replicate tissue engineering applications of the natural ECM and provide an ideal environment for cell growth and tissue regeneration. The ability to create a biomimetic environment is particularly crucial for tissue engineering since it enhances cell adhesion, differentiation, and proliferation, leading to the development of functional tissues. This section will explore various examples of peptide-based biomaterial scaffolds and hydrogels for tissue engineering applications as shown in Figure 5.4, respectively.

5.3.1.1 Bone tissue engineering

Bone tissue engineering involves the creation of bone grafts that mimic the natural bone's structure and composition. Peptide-based biomaterial scaffolds and hydrogels have been extensively researched for their potential use in bone tissue engineering. For example, researchers have developed self-assembling peptide hydrogels (SAPHs) that mimic the structure of the natural ECM and promote cell adhesion, differentiation, and proliferation.[57] For use in biomedical applications, SAPHs are a potential family of *de novo* synthetic biomaterials that combine the advantages of both natural and artificial hydrogels. These hydrogels are suitable and effective instruments to combat intervertebral disc (IVD) degeneration (one of the reasons for low back pain) due to inherent characteristics like shear-thinning behavior, excellent biocompatibility, ECM biomimicry, and tuneable physiochemical properties.[58] Furthermore, SAPHs have been used to regenerate bone tissue *in vitro* and *in vivo*, and the results have been promising.[59]

5.3.1.2 Cartilage tissue engineering

Cartilage tissue engineering involves the creation of cartilage grafts that mimic the natural cartilage's structure and composition. Peptide-based biomaterial scaffolds and hydrogels have been investigated for their potential use in cartilage tissue engineering.[60] For instance, researchers have developed a peptide hydrogel that mimics the natural ECM and promotes chondrogenic differentiation.[61] A study used Michael addition chemistry to chemically insert a collagen mimetic peptide (CMP) with the sequence (GPO)4GFOGER(GPO)4GCG into a poly(ethylene glycol) (PEG) hydrogel. The CMP contains a GFOGER sequence flanked by GPO repeat units. Human mesenchymal stem cells (hMSCs) were employed as a platform for encapsulation, proliferation, and differentiation into neocartilage/chondrocytes using the PEG/CMP hybrid hydrogel. The findings showed that, in comparison with PEG hydrogels without the peptide, PEG-CMP hydrogels offered hMSCs a natural environment that encouraged chondrogenesis and increased secretion of cartilage-specific ECM. Thus, hydrogel was found to improve the growth and proliferation of chondrocytes, leading to the regeneration of cartilage tissue.[62]

5.3.1.3 Skin tissue engineering

Skin tissue engineering encompasses the creation of skin grafts that are similar to the natural skin's structure and composition. Peptide-based biomaterial scaffolds and hydrogels have been researched for their potential use in skin tissue engineering.[62] Because they offer a three-dimensional environment and a high water content, hydrogels have gained significant attention in tissue engineering because they imitate the conditions that lead to the development of new tissue. Peptide-based hydrogels have gained increased attention as a result of their ability to mimic proteins, particularly ECM proteins, and the vast range of functions they can perform. Under the right circumstances, a noncovalent self-assembly process can be exploited to cause hydrogenation, resulting in the self-assembly of nanofibers in fiber-based hydrogels. As these fibers extend in 3D, their thickness and length increase, finally resulting in fibrillar networks. These intricate networks of peptides can trap water in this way, creating a hydrogel that can support itself.[64] An example of noncovalent interaction to create peptide-based hydrogels is the ability to create a physical hydrogel that is bioinspired and capable of healing after shearing. Shear recovery can help with bioprinting-based tissue engineering and minimally invasive techniques. Stem cell transplantation is frequently linked to low cell survival in tissue engineering. These hydrogels' characteristics allow them to be administered directly from the needle and enhance cell.[65]

5.3.1.4 Nerve tissue engineering

Nerve tissue engineering involves the creation of nerve grafts similar to natural nerve structure and composition. Peptide-based biomaterial scaffolds and hydrogels have been investigated for their potential use in nerve tissue engineering. Researchers have developed a peptide hydrogel that mimics the natural ECM and promotes nerve cell development and proliferation. As demonstrated by the self-assembly of the ionic self-complementary peptide d-EAK16, which is composed of alanine, glutamic acid, and lysine, into a nanofiber scaffold, peptide self-assembly directs the design and production of nanofiber scaffolds.[66] The hydrogel has been found to enhance axonal growth and guide the direction of nerve regeneration, leading to the development of functional nerve tissue.

5.3.1.5 Muscle tissue engineering

Muscle tissue engineering involves the creation of muscle grafts, the natural form of muscle's structure and composition. Peptide-based biomaterial scaffolds and hydrogels have been researched for their potential use in muscle tissue engineering. Researchers have developed a peptide hydrogel that mimics the natural ECM and promotes the growth and proliferation of muscle cells. Due to their correct conductivity and ability to aid in the creation of muscle tissue, conductive biomaterials make excellent candidates for use as scaffolds in muscle tissue engineering.⁶⁷ The hydrogel has been found to enhance muscle cell differentiation and fusion, leading to the development of functional muscle tissue.⁶⁸

Peptide-based biomaterial scaffolds and hydrogels have demonstrated significant promise in tissue engineering applications. They mimic the natural ECM and provide an ideal environment for cell growth and tissue regeneration. Researchers have developed various peptide-based biomaterial scaffolds and hydrogels for different tissue engineering applications, including bone, cartilage, skin, nerve, and muscle tissue engineering. The results have been promising, and peptide-based biomaterial scaffolds and hydrogels may soon become a common tool for tissue engineering applications. Further research is necessary to optimize peptide-based biomaterial scaffolds and hydrogels; however, the potential benefits for numerous tissue engineering applications are enormous.

5.4 INTRODUCTION TO PEPTIDE-BASED IMAGING AND DIAGNOSTIC

Traditional diagnostic methods often involve invasive procedures or the use of contrast agents with potential side effects.⁶⁹ Peptide-based imaging offers a promising alternative, providing a bridge between molecular biology and clinical practice. These peptides, often derived from naturally occurring proteins, can be designed or modified to exhibit a strong affinity for specific biomarkers, cell types, or tissues associated with various diseases.⁷⁰

The core principle behind peptide-based imaging lies in the selective interaction between peptides and their designated targets. When labeled with imaging agents, such as fluorescent dyes, radioactive isotopes, or nanoparticles, these peptides enable the visualization of specific molecular events or cellular structures. This level of precision allows for the identification of disease-related changes at an early stage, even before conventional symptoms manifest.⁷¹

One of the most compelling aspects of peptide-based approaches is their versatility. Peptides are tailored to target various disease markers, including overexpressed receptors on cancer cells, inflammatory molecules, and enzymes linked to neurodegenerative disorders. As a result, peptide-based imaging holds promise across diverse medical fields, spanning oncology, cardiology, neurology, and infectious diseases.⁷² As research continues to advance, the integration of peptide-based strategies into routine medical practice may significantly enhance our ability to detect diseases earlier, monitor treatment responses, and ultimately improve patient outcomes.

5.4.1 PEPTIDE-BASED IMAGING AGENTS AND PROBES FOR DISEASE DIAGNOSIS

Peptide-based imaging agents and probes are increasingly being used for disease diagnosis due to their high specificity and sensitivity. These imaging agents and probes are designed to target specific biomolecules or cells in the body and enable the detection and visualization of diseases at an early stage. Here we explore

Applications of peptide-conjugated nanomaterials 107

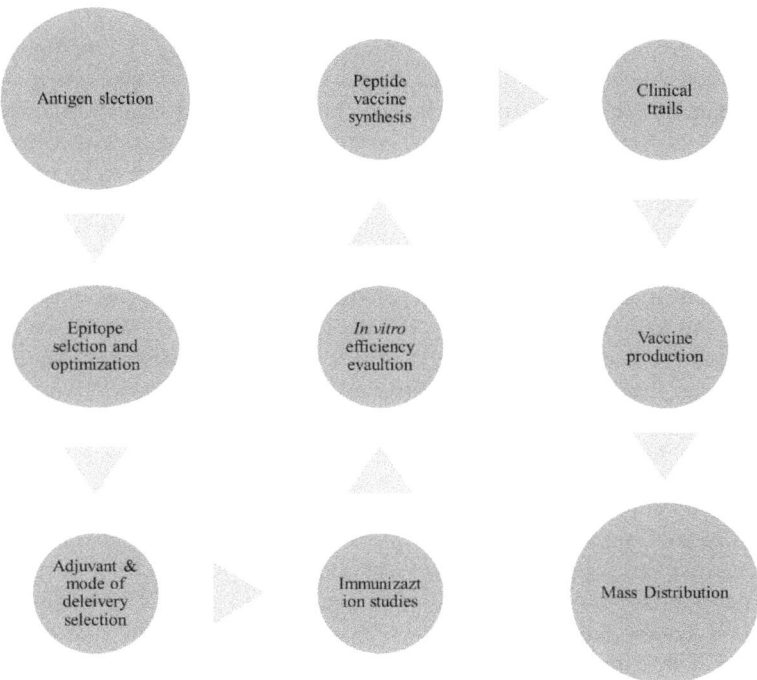

FIGURE 5.4 Peptides can self-assemble into a variety of 0D, 1D, 2D, and 3D structures. Reproduced with permission from[63]. Copyright © 2022 Elsevier.

the various examples of peptide-based imaging agents and probes for disease diagnosis.

5.4.1.1 Cancer imaging

Peptide-based imaging agents and probes are being extensively researched for their potential use in cancer imaging. For example, peptide-based radiolabeled imaging agents that selectively target cancer cells have been created. These imaging agents are designed to bind to cancer cells' surface receptors, allowing the detection and visualization of cancer cells using two imaging procedures positron emission tomography (PET) and single-photon emission computed tomography (SPECT) are two imaging procedures.[73] One example of a peptide-based imaging agent for cancer diagnosis is 68Ga-DOTA-TOC, which targets somatostatin receptors overexpressed in neuroendocrine tumors.[74] Dual-labeled with a radionuclide and fluorescent dye can get over this restriction and combine intraoperative fluorescence imaging with quantitative, whole-body nuclear imaging. IRDye 800CW was attached to the clinically utilized somatostatin analog, 68Ga-DOTA-TOC, using a multimodality chelation (MMC) scaffold to create the dual-labeled analog, 68Ga-MMC(IRDye 800CW)-TOC, with a high-yield and targeted activity.[75]

5.4.1.2 Alzheimer's disease imaging

Peptide-based imaging agents and probes are also being studied for their potential use in Alzheimer's disease diagnosis. Researchers have developed amyloid-beta (Aβ) peptide-based imaging agents that can bind to amyloid plaques in the brain, a hallmark of Alzheimer's disease.[76] These imaging agents enable the detection and visualization of amyloid plaques in the brain using imaging techniques such as PET and magnetic resonance imaging (MRI). One example of a peptide-based imaging tool for Alzheimer's disease diagnosis is 18F-NAV4694, which binds to Aβ plaques and is currently in clinical trials.[77] It has been suggested that the physiological concentration of the Aβ peptide in the brain has a role in regulating neurogenesis and synaptic plasticity. However, excessive Aβ synthesis, its aggregation, and its deposition adversely impact numerous biologically significant pathways that result in the death of neuronal cells. To prevent or treat Alzheimer's disease, research has focused on inhibiting the generation of Aβ, Aβ aggregation, or Aβ's clearance from the brain.[76]

5.4.1.3 Cardiovascular disease imaging

Peptide-based imaging agents and probes are being investigated for their potential use in cardiovascular disease diagnosis. Researchers have developed peptide-based imaging agents that can bind to specific biomolecules in the blood vessels, allowing the detection and visualization of atherosclerotic plaques.[77] These imaging agents enable the diagnosis of cardiovascular diseases at an early stage, allowing for timely interventions to prevent disease progression. One example of a peptide-based imaging agent for cardiovascular disease diagnosis is ^{99}mTc-NC100692, which targets collagen in atherosclerotic plaques,[78] and is a condition when the vessel wall develops lipid-rich atheroma. It causes a narrowing of the artery lumen, and symptomatic atherosclerosis may reduce blood flow to the subtended organs, resulting in angina or a brief ischemic event in the brain.

5.4.1.4 Inflammatory disease imaging

Peptide-based imaging agents and probes are also being studied for their potential use in inflammatory disease diagnosis. Researchers have developed peptide-based imaging agents that can bind to specific cells implementing a role in the inflammatory response, such as leukocytes and macrophages.[79] These imaging agents enable the detection and visualization of inflammation sites in the body using imaging techniques such as PET and MRI. One such example of a peptide-based imaging agent for inflammatory disease diagnosis is ^{18}F-FDG, which targets glucose uptake in activated inflammatory cells.[80]

5.4.1.5 Infectious disease imaging

Peptide-based imaging agents and probes are being investigated for their potential use in infectious disease diagnosis. Researchers have developed peptide-based imaging agents that can bind to specific infectious agents, such as bacteria and viruses. These imaging agents enable the detection and visualization of infectious agents in the body using imaging techniques such as PET and MRI. One example of a peptide-based imaging agent for infectious disease diagnosis is 99mTc-labeled ciprofloxacin, which targets bacterial infections.[70]

Peptide-based imaging agents and probes are increasingly being used for disease diagnosis due to their high specificity and sensitivity. Researchers have developed various peptide-based imaging agents and probes for various disorders, such as cancer, Alzheimer's disease, cardiovascular disease, inflammatory disease, and infectious disease. The results have been promising, and peptide-based imaging agents and probes may soon become a common tool for disease diagnosis. Further research is necessary to optimize peptide-based imaging agents and probes for various diseases, but the potential benefits are immense.

5.4.2 Peptide-based probes for imaging of biological processes

Peptide-based probes have emerged as promising tools for imaging biological processes in living systems. These probes, consisting of a peptide conjugated to a reporter molecule, can target specific biomolecules or cells, enabling the visualization of biological processes in real time. In this section, we will explore the various examples of peptide-based probes for imaging biological processes.

5.4.2.1 Cellular imaging

Peptide-based probes are being extensively researched for their potential use in cellular imaging. These probes can specific cell surface receptors or intracellular proteins which could be targeted, enabling the visualization of cellular processes such as cell signaling, apoptosis, and differentiation. One example of a peptide-based probe for cellular imaging is the RGD (Arg-Gly-Asp) peptide, which targets $\alpha v \beta 3$ integrin receptors overexpressed in cancer cells. RGD peptides have been conjugated with fluorescent dyes or radiolabels to enable the detection and visualization of cancer cells using imaging techniques such as confocal microscopy, PET, and SPECT.[81]

5.4.2.2 Neuronal imaging

Peptide-based probes are also being studied for their potential use in neuronal imaging. These probes can target specific biomolecules or cells in the nervous system, enabling the visualization of neuronal processes such as synapse formation, neurotransmitter release, and neurodegeneration. One example of a peptide-based probe for neuronal imaging is the Tat peptide, which can be permiable through the blood-brain barrier (BBB) and target neurons. Tat peptides have been conjugated with fluorescent dyes or magnetic nanoparticles to enable the detection and visualization of neurons *in vivo* using imaging techniques such as fluorescence microscopy and MRI.

5.4.2.3 Inflammation imaging

Peptide-based probes are being investigated for their potential use in inflammation imaging. These probes can target specific cells or biomolecules involved in the inflammatory response, enabling the visualization of inflammation sites in the body. One example of a peptide-based probe for inflammation imaging is the PEGylated fibrin-binding peptide, which can target fibrin deposition in inflamed tissues.[82] Fibrin-binding peptides have been conjugated with fluorescent dyes or radionuclides to enable the detection and visualization of inflammation sites *in vivo* using imaging techniques such as fluorescence microscopy, PET, and SPECT.[83]

5.4.2.4 Cardiovascular imaging

Peptide-based probes are also being studied for their potential use in cardiovascular imaging. These probes can target specific biomolecules or cells in the blood vessels, enabling the visualization of cardiovascular processes such as atherosclerosis and thrombosis. One example of a peptide-based probe for cardiovascular imaging is the cyclic RGD peptide, which can target $\alpha v \beta 3$ integrin receptors expressed in activated ECs and smooth muscle cells in atherosclerotic plaques. RGD peptides have been conjugated with fluorescent dyes or radiolabels to enable the detection and visualization of atherosclerotic plaques using imaging techniques such as fluorescence microscopy, PET, and SPECT.[83]

5.4.2.5 Metabolic imaging

Peptide-based probes are also being investigated for their potential use in metabolic imaging. These probes can target specific biomolecules or cells involved in metabolic processes, enabling the visualization of metabolic activity in living systems. One example of a peptide-based probe for metabolic imaging is the glucose-binding peptide, which can target glucose *in vivo*.[84] Glucose-binding peptides have been conjugated with fluorescent dyes or radiolabels to enable the detection and visualization of glucose uptake in living systems using imaging techniques such as fluorescence microscopy, PET, and SPECT.

Peptide-based probes have shown great potential for imaging biological processes in living systems. These probes can target specific biomolecules or cells, enabling the visualization of cellular, neuronal, inflammatory, cardiovascular, and metabolic processes in real time. The use of peptide-based probes in imaging can facilitate the understanding of complex biological processes and the discovery of novel therapies for various diseases. Further research is necessary to optimize peptide-based probes for various imaging applications, but the potential benefits of peptide-based probes for imaging biological processes are immense, and the field is continuously evolving. With further research, peptide-based probes can become even more specific and sensitive, enabling the detection and visualization of biological processes at the molecular level. One of the challenges in the advance of peptide-based probes is the optimization of their pharmacokinetics and biodistribution, to ensure that the probes reach their target sites *in vivo* and do not accumulate in nontargeted tissues. Several strategies, such as PEGylation and multivalent display, have been used to enhance the pharmacokinetics and biodistribution of peptide-based probes.

Another challenge is the selection of appropriate reporter molecules for conjugation with peptides. The reporter molecule should be able to provide high signal-to-noise ratios, have excellent photophysical properties, and be compatible with the imaging modality of choice.[85] Advances in imaging technology, such as super-resolution microscopy, may also facilitate the development of more sophisticated and specific peptide-based probes.

Peptide-based probes are a promising tool for imaging biological processes in living systems, with potential applications in disease diagnosis, drug development, and personalized medicine. These probes can target specific biomolecules or cells, enabling the visualization of cellular, neuronal, inflammatory, cardiovascular, and metabolic processes in real time. The optimization of peptide-based probes for various imaging applications is crucial to unlocking their full potential in the field of biomedicine. With further research and development, peptide-based probes could revolutionize our understanding of biological processes, leading to new diagnostic and treatment solutions for a variety of disorders.

5.5 INTRODUCTION TO PEPTIDE-BASED TARGETING OF CANCER CELLS

Cancer treatment remains a serious challenge as a result of the heterogeneity of cancer cells and their ability to evade the immune system. Traditional cancer treatments, such as chemotherapy and radiation therapy, have significant side effects and often have limited efficacy. However, peptide-based targeting of cancer cells is emerging as a promising strategy for the targeted delivery of therapeutics to cancer cells while sparing normal cells.

One of the advantages of peptide-based targeting is its potential for high selectivity and specificity. Nevertheless, peptide-based targeting of cancer cells can also be used to enhance the efficacy of immunotherapy. Immunotherapy aims to stimulate the immune system to recognize and eliminate cancer cells, but its efficacy can be limited by the immune system's ability to recognize and attack cancer cells. Peptides that mimic tumor antigens are applied to stimulate the immune system to recognize and attack cancer cells selectively. For example, the peptide NY-ESO-1 (New York esophageal squamous cell carcinoma 1) is a tumor antigen that is overexpressed in some types of cancer, including melanoma, lung cancer, and ovarian cancer. The conjugation of NY-ESO-1 peptides with dendritic cells or nanoparticles can boost the immune system's ability to detect and attack NY-ESO-1-positive cancer cells.[86]

Peptide-based targeting of cancer cells is a rapidly growing field, with potential applications in various types of cancer. The development of new peptides that selectively target cancer cells is essential for the optimization of this strategy. In addition, the optimization of peptide conjugation with various moieties, such as nanoparticles, chemotherapy drugs, or imaging agents, is crucial for enhancing the selectivity and efficacy of peptide-based targeting. Several peptide-based strategies for targeting are actively being developed in preclinical and clinical trials, including peptide-conjugated nanoparticles, peptide vaccines, and peptide-drug conjugates.

Peptide-based targeting of cancer cells is a promising strategy for the selective delivery of therapeutics to cancer cells while sparing normal cells. Peptides can selectively bind to specific receptors or antigens on the surface of cancer cells, enabling the selective imaging or treatment of cancer cells. Peptide-based targeting can also be used to enhance the efficacy of immunotherapy by stimulating the immune system to recognize and strike cancer cells. The optimization of peptide-based targeting is crucial for the development of new cancer diagnostic and treatment solutions. With further research and development, peptide-based targeting of cancer cells could revolutionize cancer treatment and improve patient outcomes.

5.5.1 Peptide-conjugated chemotherapeutic and immunotherapy agents

Peptide conjugation is establishing itself as a viable method for enhancing the efficacy and selectivity of chemotherapeutic and immunotherapy agents. Peptides can be conjugated with chemotherapeutic agents or immunotherapy agents, such as monoclonal antibodies, to enhance their delivery and selectivity to cancer cells or immune cells.

Chemotherapeutic agents, such as doxorubicin and paclitaxel, have significant side effects and often have limited efficacy due to their nonspecific distribution in the body.[87] Peptide conjugation can improve the delivery of selective chemotherapeutic toolsto cancer cells while sparing normal cells. For example, the peptide RGD targets integrin receptors, which are overexpressed on the surface of many types of cancer cells. The conjugation of RGD peptides with chemotherapeutic agents, such as paclitaxel, has been shown to improve the method of delivery of these agents to cancer cells while reducing their toxicity to normal cells.

In addition, peptide conjugation can improve the pharmacokinetic properties of chemotherapeutic agents. Peptide conjugation can improve the solubility and stability of chemotherapeutic agents, leading to improved pharmacokinetic properties and enhanced therapeutic efficacy. For example, the conjugation of the peptide PEG with chemotherapeutic agents has been shown to improve their solubility and stability, leading to improved pharmacokinetic properties and enhanced therapeutic efficacy.

Peptide conjugation can also enhance the selectivity and efficacy of immunotherapy agents. Immunotherapy agents, such as monoclonal antibodies, can target specific antigens on cancer cells or immune cells, leading to their selective destruction. Peptide conjugation can enhance the selectivity and efficacy of monoclonal antibodies by improving their affinity and specificity for their target antigens. For example, the peptide HER2 (human epidermal growth factor receptor 2) targets HER2 receptors, which are highly expressed in some breast, ovarian, and gastric cancers. The conjugation of HER2 peptides with monoclonal antibodies, such as trastuzumab, has been shown to enhance their selectivity and efficacy in HER2-positive cancer cells.

Peptide conjugation can also enhance the delivery of immunotherapy agents to immune cells. Peptides can selectively bind to specific receptors or antigens on immune cells, leading to their selective delivery. For example, the peptide

Applications of peptide-conjugated nanomaterials

TLR (toll-like receptor) targets toll-like receptors, which are discovered on the surfaces of immunological cell cells.[88] The conjugation of TLR peptides with immunotherapy agents, such as CpG oligodeoxynucleotides, has been shown to enhance their delivery to immune cells and improve their efficacy in stimulating the immune system.[89]

Moreover, *in silico* studies related to peptide inhibitors targeting cancer receptors are rapidly advancing, providing valuable insights into the stability of receptor-peptide complexes before cancer peptide drug production. This technology not only enhances our understanding of molecular interactions but also significantly reduces development costs by enabling efficient screening and optimization of potential drug candidates [90,91].

We understand peptides can selectively bind to specific receptors or antigens on cancer cells or immune cells, leading to their selective destruction or activation. Peptide conjugation can improve the pharmacokinetic properties of chemotherapeutic agents and enhance the selectivity and efficacy of immunotherapy agents. With further research and development, peptide-conjugated chemotherapeutic and immunotherapy agents could revolutionize cancer treatment and improve patient outcomes.

5.6 PEPTIDE-BASED VACCINES

5.6.1 Peptide-based Vaccines for Infectious Diseases, Cancer, Allergies, and Autoimmune Diseases

Peptide-based vaccines have emerged as a promising approach for preventing and treating infectious diseases, cancer, allergies, and autoimmune diseases. Peptide-based vaccines are designed to elicit an immune response against specific antigens, which can lead to the destruction of infectious agents or cancer cells or the suppression of immune responses in allergies and autoimmune diseases. Figure 5.5 explains the production process.

Peptide-based vaccines have been developed for several infectious diseases, including influenza, HIV, and hepatitis B and C.[92] These vaccines are designed to cause an immune system reaction against specific antigens on the surface of the infectious agents, which can cause damage to the virus or bacteria. For example, a peptide-based vaccine for hepatitis B has been developed that targets the hepatitis B surface antigen. This vaccine has been shown to be effective in preventing hepatitis B infection and is currently being used in many countries as part of routine vaccination programs. Epitope prediction is an important step in this process (Figure 5.4). An epitope (or antigenic determinant) is a component of the antigen that immune cells recognize, consisting of 5–15 amino acid residues or 1–6 sugar residues. The T and B cells mediate cellular and humoral immunological pathways in the adaptive immune system. These immune cells may recognize previously encountered immunogenic epitopes, eliciting a rapid and long-lasting immunological response that serves as the foundation for vaccination.[92]

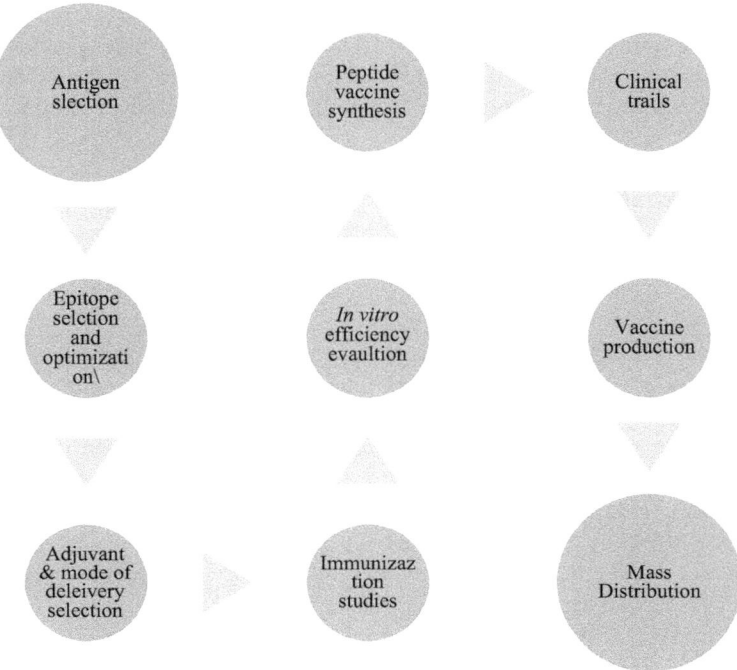

FIGURE 5.5 A schematic representation of the vaccine development process.

In cancer, peptide-based vaccines have also been developed to induce an immune response against cancer-specific antigens. These vaccines can stimulate the immune system to recognize and attack cancer cells, leading to their destruction. For example, a peptide-based vaccine for PCa has been developed that targets the PSA.[93] This vaccination has been scientifically proven to improve survival in patients with advanced PCa by inducing an immune response to PSA. The most widely employed blood cancer marker is PSA, an androgenregulated serine protease generated by both prostatic epithelial cells and PCa. It refers to the tissue kallikrein family, which includes some members whichare likewise prostate-specific. PSA is a key protein in sperm, where it cleaves semenogelins in the seminal coagulum. It is released into the prostatic ducts as an inactive 244-amino acid proenzyme (proPSA), which is triggered by the cleavage of seven N-terminal amino acids. PSA that enters the bloodstream unbound is immediately absorbed by protease inhibitors., notably alpha1-antichymotrypsin; however, a proportion is inactivated by proteolysis in the lumen and circulates as free PSA.[94]

To suppress immune responses to allergens, peptide-based vaccines have also been developed for allergies. These vaccines are designed to induce tolerance to specific allergens, which can prevent allergic reactions. For example, a peptide-based vaccine for ragweed allergy has been developed that targets a specific region of the ragweed allergen.[95] This vaccine has been shown to induce tolerance to ragweed and to reduce symptoms of ragweed allergy.

Vaccines based on peptides were additionally created for autoimmune diseases to suppress immune responses against self-antigens. These vaccines are designed to induce tolerance to specific self-antigens, which can prevent autoimmune attacks. For example, a peptide-based vaccine for type 1 diabetes has been developed that targets the insulin B chain. This vaccine has been shown to induce tolerance to the insulin B chain and to delay the onset of type 1 diabetes in animal models.[96] Insulin B chain peptide 9–23 (B: 9–23; SHLVEALYLVCGERG) and its analogs have been demonstrated as well to prevent nonobese diabetic (NOD) mice from diabetes. Thus, Eisenbarth *et al.* established the effectiveness of administering an equivalent of insulin B: 9–23 peptide (the Cytotoxic T Lymphocyte (CTL) sequence was truncated) to NOD mice (20 g/administration starting at four weeks of age, and administered at days 1–5 and 8, and then every week until 10 weeks of age). This resulted in the elimination of spontaneous insulin autoantibodies, considerable suppression of insulitis, and recovery from the hyperglycemia.[97] In a mouse model of RA, vaccination with a biologically inactive but immunogenic human TNF derivative [keyhole limpet hemocyanin (KLH)-human TNF heterocomplex] resulted in high levels of neutralizing antibodies and defense against arthritis.[98]

Nevertheless, peptide-based vaccines have several advantages over traditional vaccines, including improved safety, specificity, and stability. Peptide-based vaccines are less likely to cause adverse reactions or to induce immune responses against nontarget antigens. Peptide-based vaccines can also be designed to target specific regions of antigens, which can improve their specificity and reduce the risk of cross-reactivity with nontarget antigens. Finally, peptide-based vaccines are more stable than traditional vaccines, which can reduce the need for cold storage and transportation.

Peptide-based vaccines have emerged as a promising approach for preventing and treating infectious diseases, cancer, allergies, and autoimmune diseases. Peptide-based vaccines can induce immune responses against specific antigens, leading to the destruction of infectious agents or cancer cells, or the suppression of immune responses in allergies and autoimmune diseases. With further research and development, peptide-based vaccines could revolutionize the prevention and treatment of many diseases, improving patient outcomes and quality of life.

5.6.2 Peptide-conjugated Chemotherapeutic and Immunotherapy Agents

Peptide-conjugated chemotherapeutic and immunotherapy agents recently emerged as an alternative to therapy for cancer and other disorders. These agents are designed to specifically target cancer cells or other disease targets while sparing healthy cells, which can reduce the risk of adverse side effects associated with traditional chemotherapy and immunotherapy.

Chemotherapeutic agents are based on peptides designed to specifically deliver drugs specifically to cancer cells, which can increase the efficacy of the drug while reducing its toxicity to healthy cells. For example, a peptide-conjugated doxorubicin has been developed that targets the αvβ3 integrin, which is found on the outermost layer of many various kinds of cancer cells. This peptide-conjugated doxorubicin has been shown to be more effective at killing cancer cells and reducing tumor growth than traditional doxorubicin while causing fewer side effects.[99] Because integrin αvβ3 plays a critical role due to its affinity for the RGD sequence, which is known to accumulates in cancer and endothelial cells, numerous nanocarriers for using RGD for tumor identification, drug carriers, or boosting RGD therapeutic impact have been developed. RGD sequences connected with molybdenum dioxide (MoS_2)/gadolinium (Gd) including RGD sequences were used for cancer MRI. The MoS_2-Gd-RGD nanoparticles demonstrated integrin v3 targeting properties in in vitro and in vivo research. Thus, MoS_2-Gd-RGD nanoparticles have the potential to be used as MR contrast agents.[100]

Peptide-conjugated immunotherapy agents are designed to stimulate the immune system to specifically target cancer cells or other disease targets. For example, a peptide-conjugated monoclonal antibody has been developed that targets the CD20 antigen on the surface of B-cell lymphoma cells. This peptide-conjugated antibody has been shown to be more effective at inducing immune responses against B-cell lymphoma cells than traditional monoclonal antibodies, leading to improved patient outcomes.[101] CD20 expression is restricted to precursor B cells, mature B cells, and the majority of neoplastic B cells from (Non-Hodgkin Lymphoma) NHL patients, all of which have high concentrations of CD20 on their cell surface.[102]

As discussed earlier, peptide-conjugated chemotherapeutic and immunotherapy agents have several advantages over traditional chemotherapy and immunotherapy. Peptide-conjugated agents can be designed to specifically target cancer cells or other disease targets, which can increase their efficacy while reducing their toxicity to healthy cells. Peptide-conjugated agents can also be designed to be more stable and have longer half-lives than traditional drugs, which can reduce the need for frequent dosing. Additionally, peptide-conjugated agents can be designed to be more easily internalized by cancer cells, which can increase their effectiveness at killing cancer cells.

Despite the promising potential of peptide-conjugated chemotherapeutic and immunotherapy agents, there are several challenges that must be addressed before they can become widely used in clinical practice. One of the challenges is the need for better methods of targeting cancer cells or other disease targets with high specificity. Another challenge is the need to optimize the pharmacokinetics and pharmacodynamics of peptide-conjugated agents to maximize their efficacy while minimizing their toxicity to healthy cells. Finally, there is a need for further research to understand the mechanisms of action of peptide-conjugated agents, which can exhibit the production of new and more effective treatments.

Peptide-conjugated chemotherapeutic and immunotherapy agents have appeared as promising approaches for the treatment of cancer and other diseases. These agents can be created especially to target cancer cells or other disease targets, which can increase their efficacy while reducing their toxicity to healthy cells. With further research and development, peptide-conjugated agents could revolutionize the treatment of many diseases, improving patient outcomes and quality of life.

5.7 PRACTICAL QUESTIONS

1. What are some specific biomedical applications where peptides conjugated to nanomaterials have shown significant promise, and how do these applications leverage the unique properties of both components?
2. Can you elaborate on the mechanisms by which peptides enhance the targeting and internalization of nanomaterials into specific cell types or tissues?
3. In the context of cancer therapy, how do peptide-conjugated nanomaterials contribute to improved drug delivery and reduced off-target effects?
4. What role do peptides play in stabilizing and functionalizing nanomaterials, and how does this influence their overall performance in various applications?
5. Could you provide examples of recent advancements or breakthroughs in the field of diagnostics that have been achieved through the utilization of peptides conjugated with nanomaterials?

REFERENCES

1. Smith, T. T.; Stephan, S. B.; Moffett, H. F.; McKnight, L. E.; Ji, W.; Reiman, D.; Bonagofski, E.; Wohlfahrt, M. E.; Pillai, S. P. S.; Stephan, M. T., In situ programming of leukaemia-specific T cells using synthetic DNA nanocarriers. *Nature Nanotechnology* 2017, 12 (8), 813–820.
2. Bharali, D. J.; Lucey, D. W.; Jayakumar, H.; Pudavar, H. E.; Prasad, P. N., Folate-receptor-mediated delivery of InP quantum dots for bioimaging using confocal and two-photon microscopy. *Journal of the American Chemical Society* 2005, 127 (32), 11364–11371.
3. Salerno, M.; Santo Domingo Porqueras, D., Alzheimer's disease: The use of contrast agents for magnetic resonance imaging to detect amyloid beta peptide inside the brain. *Coordination Chemistry Reviews* 2016, 327–328, 27–34.
4. Senapati, S.; Mahanta, A. K.; Kumar, S.; Maiti, P., Controlled drug delivery vehicles for cancer treatment and their performance. *Signal Transduction and Targeted Therapy* 2018, 3 (1), 7.
5. Liu, Q.; Wang, J.; Boyd, B. J., Peptide-based biosensors. *Talanta* 2015, 136, 114–127.

6. Babitha, S.; Annamalai, M.; Dykas, M. M.; Saha, S.; Poddar, K.; Venugopal, J. R.; Ramakrishna, S.; Venkatesan, T.; Korrapati, P. S., Fabrication of a biomimetic ZeinPDA nanofibrous scaffold impregnated with BMP-2 peptide conjugated TiO_2 nanoparticle for bone tissue engineering. *Journal of Tissue Engineering and Regenerative Medicine* 2018, *12* (4), 991–1001.
7. Liang, J.; Mazur, F.; Tang, C.; Ning, X.; Chandrawati, R.; Liang, K., Peptide-induced super-assembly of biocatalytic metal–organic frameworks for programmed enzyme cascades. *Chemical Science* 2019, 10 (34), 7852–7858.
8. Shen, Y.; Cao, B.; Snyder, N. R.; Woeppel, K. M.; Eles, J. R.; Cui, X. T., ROS responsive resveratrol delivery from LDLR peptide conjugated PLA-coated mesoporous silica nanoparticles across the blood–brain barrier. *Journal of Nanobiotechnology* 2018, 16 (1), 13.
9. Zheng, X. T.; Tan, Y. N., Recent development of nucleic acid nanosensors to detect sequence-specific binding interactions: From metal ions, small molecules to proteins and pathogens. *Sensors International* 2020, *1*, 100034.
10. Bhakta, S.; Mishra, P., Molecularly imprinted polymer-based sensors for cancer biomarker detection. *Sensors and Actuators Reports* 2021, *3*, 100061.
11. Yuan, L.; Liu, L., Peptide-based electrochemical biosensing. *Sensors and Actuators B: Chemical* 2021, *344*, 130232.
12. Pröll, F., Biosensors 2008—The tenth world congress on biosensors. *Analytical and Bioanalytical Chemistry* 2008, 392 (7), 1257–1259.
13. Borisov, S. M.; Wolfbeis, O. S., Optical biosensors. *Chemical Reviews* 2008, 108 (2), 423–461.
14. Fan, X.; White, I. M.; Shopova, S. I.; Zhu, H.; Suter, J. D.; Sun, Y., Sensitive optical biosensors for unlabeled targets: A review. *Analytica Chimica Acta* 2008, 620 (1), 8–26.
15. Liu, Q.; Wang, J.; Boyd, B. J., Peptide-based biosensors. *Talanta* 2015, 136, 114–27.
16. Guo, X., Surface plasmon resonance based biosensor technique: A review. *Journal of Biophotonics* 2012, 5 (7), 483–501.
17. Sharma, S.; Kumari, R.; Varshney, S. K.; Lahiri, B., Optical biosensing with electromagnetic nanostructures. *Reviews in Physics* 2020, 5, 100044.
18. Guo, X., Surface plasmon resonance based biosensor technique: A review. *Journal of Biophotonics* 2012, 5 (7), 483–501.
19. Jacobs, C. B.; Peairs, M. J.; Venton, B. J., Review: Carbon nanotube based electrochemical sensors for biomolecules. *Analytica Chimica Acta* 2010, 662 (2), 105–127.
20. Huang, W.; Diallo, A. K.; Dailey, J. L.; Besar, K.; Katz, H. E., Electrochemical processes and mechanistic aspects of field-effect sensors for biomolecules. *Journal of Materials Chemistry* C 2015, 3 (25), 6445–6470.
21. Vanova, V.; Mitrevska, K.; Milosavljevic, V.; Hynek, D.; Richtera, L.; Adam, V., Peptide-based electrochemical biosensors utilized for protein detection. *Biosensors and Bioelectronics* 2021, 180, 113087.
22. Zhang, Y.; Wang, Y.; Guan, Y.; Zhang, Y., Peptide-enhanced tough, resilient and adhesive eutectogels for highly reliable strain/pressure sensing under extreme conditions. *Nature Communications* 2022, 13 (1), 6671.
23. Cheng, Y.; Koh, L.-D.; Li, D.; Ji, B.; Zhang, Y.; Yeo, J.; Guan, G.; Han, M.-Y.; Zhang, Y.-W., Peptide–graphene interactions enhance the mechanical properties of silk fibroin. *ACS Applied Materials & Interfaces* 2015, 7 (39), 21787–21796.
24. George Kerry, R.; Ukhurebor, K. E.; Kumari, S.; Maurya, G. K.; Patra, S.; Panigrahi, B.; Majhi, S.; Rout, J. R.; Rodriguez-Torres, M. d. P.; Das, G.; Shin, H.-S.; Patra, J. K., A comprehensive review on the applications of nano-biosensor-based approaches for non-communicable and communicable disease detection. *Biomaterials Science* 2021, *9* (10), 3576–3602.

25. Guida, F.; Battisti, A.; Gladich, I.; Buzzo, M.; Marangon, E.; Giodini, L.; Toffoli, G.; Laio, A.; Berti, F., Peptide biosensors for anticancer drugs: Design in silico to work in denaturing environment. *Biosensors and Bioelectronics* 2018, 100, 298–303.
26. Ripp, S.; DiClaudio, M. L.; Sayler, G. S., Biosensors as environmental monitors. In *Environmental microbiology*, Ralph, M.; Ji-Dong, G., Eds. John Wiley & Sons, Nature: 2009; pp. 213–233.
27. Kadam, U. S.; Hong, J. C., Advances in aptameric biosensors designed to detect toxic contaminants from food, water, human fluids, and the environment. *Trends in Environmental Analytical Chemistry* 2022, *36*, e00184.
28. Latosinska, A.; Siwy, J.; Faguer, S.; Beige, J.; Mischak, H.; Schanstra, J. P., Value of urine peptides in assessing kidney and cardiovascular disease. *PROTEOMICS – Clinical Applications* 2021, *15* (1), 2000027.
29. Qi, H.; Li, M.; Dong, M.; Ruan, S.; Gao, Q.; Zhang, C., Electrogenerated chemiluminescence peptide-based biosensor for the determination of prostate-specific antigen based on target-induced cleavage of peptide. *Analytical Chemistry* 2014, 86 (3), 1372–1379.
30. Shayesteh, O. H.; Ghavami, R., A novel label-free colorimetric aptasensor for sensitive determination of PSA biomarker using gold nanoparticles and a cationic polymer in human serum. *Spectrochimica Acta Part A: Molecular and Biomolecular Spectroscopy* 2020, 226, 117644.
31. Bergström, G.; Mandenius, C.-F., Orientation and capturing of antibody affinity ligands: Applications to surface plasmon resonance biochips. *Sensors and Actuators B: Chemical* 2011, *158* (1), 265–270.
32. Verma, N.; Kaur, G., Chapter 8-advances in the oligonucleotide-based biosensors for the detection of heavy metal contaminants in the environment. In *Tools, techniques and protocols for monitoring environmental contaminants*, Kaur Brar, S.; Hegde, K.; Pachapur, V. L., Eds. Elsevier: 2019; pp. 169–185.
33. Tsopela, A.; Laborde, A.; Salvagnac, L.; Ventalon, V.; Bedel-Pereira, E.; Séguy, I.; Temple-Boyer, P.; Juneau, P.; Izquierdo, R.; Launay, J., Development of a lab-on-chip electrochemical biosensor for water quality analysis based on microalgal photosynthesis. *Biosensors and Bioelectronics* 2016, 79, 568–573.
34. Ejeian, F.; Etedali, P.; Mansouri-Tehrani, H.-A.; Soozanipour, A.; Low, Z.-X.; Asadnia, M.; Taheri-Kafrani, A.; Razmjou, A., Biosensors for wastewater monitoring: A review. *Biosensors and Bioelectronics* 2018, 118, 66–79.
35. Zhu, Z., An overview of carbon nanotubes and graphene for biosensing applications. *Nano-Micro Letters* 2017, *9* (3), 25.
36. Viirlaid, E.; Ilisson, M.; Kopanchuk, S.; Mäeorg, U.; Rinken, A.; Rinken, T., Immunoassay for rapid on-site detection of glyphosate herbicide. *Environmental Monitoring and Assessment* 2019, *191* (8), 507.
37. Tertis, M.; Hosu, O.; Feier, B.; Cernat, A.; Florea, A.; Cristea, C., Electrochemical peptide-based sensors for foodborne pathogens detection. *Molecules* 2021, *26* (11), 3200.
38. Qiao, Z.; Fu, Y.; Lei, C.; Li, Y., Advances in antimicrobial peptides-based biosensing methods for detection of foodborne pathogens: A review. *Food Control* 2020, *112*, 107116.
39. Denyes, J. M.; Dunne, M.; Steiner, S.; Mittelviefhaus, M.; Weiss, A.; Schmidt, H.; Klumpp, J.; Loessner, M. J., Modified bacteriophage S16 long tail fiber proteins for rapid and specific immobilization and detection of Salmonella cells. *Applied and Environmental Microbiology* 2017, *83* (12), e00277-17.
40. Homola, J., Surface plasmon resonance sensors for detection of chemical and biological species. *Chemical Reviews* 2008, 108 (2), 462–493.

41. Lee, S. J.; Yoo, J. J.; Atala, A., Biomaterials and tissue engineering. *Clinical Regenerative Medicine in Urology* 2018, 17–51.
42. Kim, T. G.; Shin, H.; Lim, D. W., Biomimetic scaffolds for tissue engineering. *Advanced Functional Materials* 2012, *22* (12), 2446–2468.
43. Arslan, E.; Garip, I. C.; Gulseren, G.; Tekinay, A. B.; Guler, M. O., Bioactive supramolecular peptide nanofibers for regenerative medicine. *Advanced Healthcare Materials* 2014, *3* (9), 1357–1376.
44. Hellman, K. B.; Johnson, P. C.; Bertram, T. A.; Tawil, B., *Challenges in tissue engineering and regenerative medicine product commercialization: Building an industry*. Mary Ann Liebert, Inc.: 2011; Vol. 17, pp. 1–3.
45. D'Andrea, L. D.; Del Gatto, A.; Pedone, C.; Benedetti, E., Peptide-based molecules in angiogenesis. *Chemical Biology & Drug Design* 2006, *67* (2), 115–126.
46. Carmeliet, P., Angiogenesis in health and disease. *Nature Medicine* 2003, *9* (6), 653–660.
47. Hanahan, D.; Folkman, J., Patterns and emerging mechanisms of the angiogenic switch during tumorigenesis. *Cell* 1996, *86* (3), 353–364.
48. D'Andrea, L. D.; Del Gatto, A.; Pedone, C.; Benedetti, E., Peptide-based molecules in angiogenesis. *Chemical Biology & Drug Design* 2006, *67* (2), 115–126.
49. Huang, G.; Li, F.; Zhao, X.; Ma, Y.; Li, Y.; Lin, M.; Jin, G.; Lu, T. J.; Genin, G. M.; Xu, F., Functional and biomimetic materials for engineering of the three-dimensional cell microenvironment. *Chemical Reviews* 2017, *117* (20), 12764–12850.
50. Veeman, D.; Sai, M. S.; Sureshkumar, P.; Jagadeesha, T.; Natrayan, L.; Ravichandran, M.; Mammo, W. D., Additive manufacturing of biopolymers for tissue engineering and regenerative medicine: An overview, potential applications, advancements, and trends. *International Journal of Polymer Science* 2021, *2021*, 1–20.
51. Castillo Diaz, L. A.; Saiani, A.; Gough, J. E.; Miller, A. F., Human osteoblasts within soft peptide hydrogels promote mineralisation in vitro. *Journal of Tissue Engineering* 2014, *5*, 2041731414539344.
52. Sordi, M. B.; Cruz, A.; Fredel, M. C.; Magini, R.; Sharpe, P. T., Three-dimensional bioactive hydrogel-based scaffolds for bone regeneration in implant dentistry. *Materials Science and Engineering:* C 2021, *124*, 112055.
53. TortelliA, F.; Cancedda, R., Three-dimensional cultures of osteogenic and chondrogenic cells: A tissue engineering approach to mimic bone and cartilage in vitro. *European Cells & Materials* 2009, *17*, 1–14.
54. Vasir, J. K.; Labhasetwar, V., Biodegradable nanoparticles for cytosolic delivery of therapeutics. *Advanced Drug Delivery Reviews* 2007, *59* (8), 718–728.
55. Eskandari, S.; Guerin, T.; Toth, I.; Stephenson, R. J., Recent advances in self-assembled peptides: Implications for targeted drug delivery and vaccine engineering. *Advanced Drug Delivery Reviews* 2017, *110*, 169–187.
56. Niidome, T.; Huang, L., Gene therapy progress and prospects: Nonviral vectors. *Gene Therapy* 2002, *9* (24), 1647–1652.
57. Wang, R.; Wang, Y.; Yang, H.; Zhao, C.; Pan, J., Research progress of self-assembling peptide hydrogels in repairing cartilage defects. *Frontiers in Materials* 2022, *9*, 1022386.
58. Ligorio, C.; Hoyland, J. A.; Saiani, A., Self-assembling peptide hydrogels as functional tools to tackle intervertebral disc degeneration. *Gels* 2022, *8* (4), 211.
59. Li, L.; Li, J.; Guo, J.; Zhang, H.; Zhang, X.; Yin, C.; Wang, L.; Zhu, Y.; Yao, Q., 3D molecularly functionalized cell-free biomimetic scaffolds for osteochondral regeneration. *Advanced Functional Materials* 2019, *29* (6), 1807356.
60. Hastar, N.; Arslan, E.; Guler, M. O.; Tekinay, A. B., Peptide-based materials for cartilage tissue regeneration. *Peptides and Peptide-Based Biomaterials and Their Biomedical Applications* 2017, *1030*, 155–166.

61. Lee, H. J.; Yu, C.; Chansakul, T.; Hwang, N. S.; Varghese, S.; Yu, S. M.; Elisseeff, J. H., Enhanced chondrogenesis of mesenchymal stem cells in collagen mimetic peptide-mediated microenvironment. *Tissue Engineering Part A* 2008, 14 (11), 1843–1851.
62. Liu, S. Q.; Tian, Q.; Hedrick, J. L.; Po Hui, J. H.; Rachel Ee, P. L.; Yang, Y. Y., Biomimetic hydrogels for chondrogenic differentiation of human mesenchymal stem cells to neocartilage. *Biomaterials* 2010, 31 (28), 7298–7307.
63. Byakodi, M.; Shrikrishna, N. S.; Sharma, R.; Bhansali, S.; Mishra, Y.; Kaushik, A.; Gandhi, S., Emerging 0D, 1D, 2D, and 3D nanostructures for efficient point-of-care biosensing. *Biosensors and Bioelectronics: X* 2022, 12, 100284.
64. Dasgupta, A.; Mondal, J. H.; Das, D., Peptide hydrogels. *RSC Advances* 2013, 3 (24), 9117–9149.
65. Bakhtiary, N.; Ghalandari, B.; Ghorbani, F.; Varma, S. N.; Liu, C., Advances in peptide-based hydrogel for tissue engineering. *Polymers* 2023, 15 (5), 1068.
66. He, B.; Yuan, X.; Jiang, D., Molecular self-assembly guides the fabrication of peptide nanofiber scaffolds for nerve repair. *RSC Advances* 2014, 4 (45), 23610–23621.
67. Dong, R.; Ma, P. X.; Guo, B., Conductive biomaterials for muscle tissue engineering. *Biomaterials* 2020, 229, 119584.
68. Holmes, T. C., Novel peptide-based biomaterial scaffolds for tissue engineering. *Trends in Biotechnology* 2002, 20 (1), 16–21.
69. Castro, D. C.; Walker, I.; Glocker, B., Causality matters in medical imaging. *Nature Communications* 2020, 11 (1), 3673.
70. Lee, S.; Xie, J.; Chen, X., Peptide-based probes for targeted molecular imaging. *Biochemistry* 2010, 49 (7), 1364–1376.
71. Lee, S.; Xie, J.; Chen, X., Peptides and peptide hormones for molecular imaging and disease diagnosis. *Chemical Reviews* 2010, 110 (5), 3087–3111.
72. James, M. L.; Gambhir, S. S., A molecular imaging primer: Modalities, imaging agents, and applications. *Physiological Reviews* 2012, 92 (2), 897–965.
73. Blake, P.; Johnson, B.; VanMeter, J. W., Positron emission tomography (PET) and single photon emission computed tomography (SPECT): Clinical applications. *Journal of Neuro-Ophthalmology* 2003, 23 (1), 34–41.
74. Gabriel, M.; Decristoforo, C.; Kendler, D.; Dobrozemsky, G.; Heute, D.; Uprimny, C.; Kovacs, P.; Von Guggenberg, E.; Bale, R.; Virgolini, I. J., 68Ga-DOTA-Tyr3-octreotide PET in neuroendocrine tumors: Comparison with somatostatin receptor scintigraphy and CT. *Journal of Nuclear Medicine* 2007, 48 (4), 508–518.
75. Ghosh, S. C.; Hernandez Vargas, S.; Rodriguez, M.; Kossatz, S.; Voss, J.; Carmon, K. S.; Reiner, T.; Schonbrunn, A.; Azhdarinia, A., Synthesis of a fluorescently labeled 68Ga-DOTA-TOC analog for somatostatin receptor targeting. *ACS Medicinal Chemistry Letters* 2017, 8 (7), 720–725.
76. Rajasekhar, K.; Chakrabarti, M.; Govindaraju, T., Function and toxicity of amyloid beta and recent therapeutic interventions targeting amyloid beta in Alzheimer's disease. *Chemical Communications* 2015, 51 (70), 13434–13450.
77. Baig, M. H.; Ahmad, K.; Rabbani, G.; Choi, I., Use of peptides for the management of Alzheimer's disease: Diagnosis and inhibition. *Frontiers in Aging Neuroscience* 2018, 10, 21.
78. Lee, S. J.; Paeng, J. C., Nuclear molecular imaging for vulnerable atherosclerotic plaques. *Korean Journal of Radiology* 2015, 16 (5), 955–966.
79. Conde, J.; Bao, C.; Tan, Y.; Cui, D.; Edelman, E. R.; Azevedo, H. S.; Byrne, H. J.; Artzi, N.; Tian, F., Dual targeted immunotherapy via in vivo delivery of biohybrid RNAi-peptide nanoparticles to tumor-associated macrophages and cancer cells. *Advanced Functional Materials* 2015, 25 (27), 4183–4194.

80. Meller, J.; Sahlmann, C.-O.; Scheel, A. K., 18F-FDG PET and PET/CT in fever of unknown origin. *Journal of Nuclear Medicine* 2007, 48 (1), 35–45.
81. Wang, C.; Chen, B.; Zou, M.; Cheng, G., Cyclic RGD-modified chitosan/graphene oxide polymers for drug delivery and cellular imaging. *Colloids and Surfaces B: Biointerfaces* 2014, 122, 332–340.
82. Liang, M.-S.; Andreadis, S. T., Engineering fibrin-binding TGF-β1 for sustained signaling and contractile function of MSC based vascular constructs. *Biomaterials* 2011, *32* (33), 8684–8693.
83. Zhou, Z.; Lu, Z.-R., Molecular imaging of the tumor microenvironment. *Advanced Drug Delivery Reviews* 2017, 113, 24–48.
84. Kassem, S.; McPhee, S. A.; Berisha, N.; Ulijn, R. V., Emergence of cooperative glucose-binding networks in adaptive peptide systems. *Journal of the American Chemical Society* 2023, 145 (17), 9800–9807.
85. Edelstein, W.; Glover, G.; Hardy, C.; Redington, R., The intrinsic signal-to-noise ratio in NMR imaging. *Magnetic Resonance in Medicine* 1986, 3 (4), 604–618.
86. Chen, J.-L.; Dunbar, P.; Gileadi, U.; Jäger, E.; Gnjatic, S.; Nagata, Y.; Stockert, E.; Panicali, D. L.; Chen, Y.-T.; Knuth, A., Identification of NY-ESO-1 peptide analogues capable of improved stimulation of tumor-reactive CTL. *The Journal of Immunology* 2000, 165 (2), 948–955.
87. Perez, E. A., Doxorubicin and paclitaxel in the treatment of advanced breast cancer: Efficacy and cardiac considerations. *Cancer Investigation* 2001, *19* (2), 155–164.
88. Dowling, J. K.; Mansell, A., Toll-like receptors: The swiss army knife of immunity and vaccine development. *Clinical & Translational Immunology* 2016, *5* (5), e85.
89. Iwasaki, A.; Medzhitov, R., Toll-like receptor control of the adaptive immune responses. *Nature Immunology* 2004, 5 (10), 987–995.
90. Senapathi, T.; Selvaraj, S.; Weerasinghe, L. A Computational Approach to Determine the Potential Inhibition of the Gomesin Peptide as an AKT1 Inhibitor in Breast Cancer 2023.
91. Anbarasu, K.; Jayanthi, S. Designing and optimization of novel human LMTK3 inhibitors against breast cancer – a computational approach. *Journal of Receptors and Signal Transduction*, 2016, 37 (1), 51–59. https://doi.org/10.3109/10799893.2016.1155069
92. Kalita, P.; Tripathi, T., Methodological advances in the design of peptide-based vaccines. *Drug Discovery Today* 2022, 27 (5), 1367–1380.
93. Balk, S. P.; Ko, Y.-J.; Bubley, G. J., Biology of prostate-specific antigen. *Journal of Clinical Oncology* 2003, 21 (2), 383–391.
94. Partin, A. W.; Catalona, W. J.; Southwick, P. C.; Subong, E. N.; Gasior, G. H.; Chan, D. W., Analysis of percent free prostate-specific antigen (PSA) for prostate cancer detection: Influence of total PSA, prostate volume, and age. *Urology* 1996, *48* (6), 55–61.
95. Alexander, C.; Kay, A. B.; Larché, M., Peptide-based vaccines in the treatment of specific allergy. *Current Drug Targets-Inflammation & Allergy* 2002, *1* (4), 353–361.
96. Fierabracci, A., Peptide immunotherapies in Type 1 diabetes: Lessons from animal models. *Current Medicinal Chemistry* 2011, 18 (4), 577–586.
97. Kobayashi, M.; Abiru, N.; Arakawa, T.; Fukushima, K.; Zhou, H.; Kawasaki, E.; Yamasaki, H.; Liu, E.; Miao, D.; Wong, F. S., Altered B: 9–23 insulin, when administered intranasally with cholera toxin adjuvant, suppresses the expression of insulin autoantibodies and prevents diabetes. *The Journal of Immunology* 2007, *179* (4), 2082–2088.

98. Le Buanec, H.; Delavallée, L.; Bessis, N.; Paturance, S.; Bizzini, B.; Gallo, R.; Zagury, D.; Boissier, M.-C., TNFα kinoid vaccination-induced neutralizing antibodies to TNFα protect mice from autologous TNFα-driven chronic and acute inflammation. *Proceedings of the National Academy of Sciences* 2006, 103 (51), 19442–19447.
99. Mulgrew, K.; Kinneer, K.; Yao, X.-T.; Ward, B. K.; Damschroder, M. M.; Walsh, B.; Mao, S.-Y.; Gao, C.; Kiener, P. A.; Coats, S., Direct targeting of αvβ3 integrin on tumor cells with a monoclonal antibody, Abegrin™. *Molecular Cancer Therapeutics* 2006, 5 (12), 3122–3129.
100. Eldar-Boock, A.; Blau, R.; Ryppa, C.; Baabur-Cohen, H.; Many, A.; Vicent, M. J.; Kratz, F.; Sanchis, J.; Satchi-Fainaro, R., Integrin-targeted nano-sized polymeric systems for paclitaxel conjugation: A comparative study. *Journal of Drug Targeting* 2017, 25 (9–10), 829–844.
101. Eisenberg, R.; Looney, R. J., The therapeutic potential of anti-CD20: "what do B-cells do?". *Clinical Immunology* 2005, 117 (3), 207–213.
102. Kunala, S.; Macklis, R. M., Ionizing radiation induces CD20 surface expression on human B cells. *International Journal of Cancer* 2001, 96 (3), 178–181.

6 Future directions and challenges in peptide nanotechnology

6.1 INTRODUCTION

Peptide nanotechnology is an evolving field that has the potential to develop many areas of science and technology; hence, researchers explore this usage to obtain novel materials and devices for the future. In recent times, many advanced applications have been present in the therapeutic field such as the usage of therapeutic agents helping to target specific cells or tissues in the body with high specificity and efficiency. Peptide-based drugs have been developed for the treatment of cancer, diabetes, and other diseases; such drugs also provide new possibilities for drug delivery to be transmitted to targeted sites in the body with high specificity and control.

Another area where peptide nanotechnology is showing great promise is in the development of new materials. Peptides can be used to create self-assembling materials, where the peptides spontaneously organize themselves into complex structures. These materials have a wide range of potential applications, from drug delivery to tissue engineering to electronics. For example, peptide-based hydrogels have been developed that can be used to regenerate damaged tissues, while peptide-based sensors have been created that can detect specific molecules with high sensitivity and specificity.

Despite the exciting potential of peptide nanotechnology, many challenges must be overcome to fully realize its potential. One of the biggest challenges is in the design and synthesis of peptides themselves. Peptides are complex molecules that can have a wide range of properties, and designing peptides that have the desired properties for a particular application can be difficult. In addition, synthesizing peptides can be a time-consuming and expensive process, making it difficult to scale up the production of peptide-based materials and devices.

We understand that peptides can form complex structures that can be difficult to analyze using traditional characterization techniques, such as microscopy or spectroscopy. New techniques and tools will be needed to fully understand the properties and behavior of peptide-based materials and devices. There is also a need for a better understanding of the interactions between peptides and biological systems. Peptides can interact with cells and tissues in complex ways, and understanding these interactions will be critical for the development of safe and effective peptide-based therapies. In addition, there is a need for a better understanding of the environmental impact of peptide-based materials and devices, and how they can be safely disposed of or recycled.

To address these challenges, researchers in peptide nanotechnology are exploring new approaches and techniques. For example, advances in computational modeling and simulation are making it possible to design peptides with specific properties and to simulate the behavior of peptide-based materials and devices. New analytical techniques, such as cryo-electron microscopy, are also allowing researchers to study the complex structures of peptide-based materials in greater detail.

In addition, researchers are exploring new ways to synthesize peptides, such as using biotechnology techniques to produce peptides in living cells or using microfluidic systems to rapidly synthesize and screen large numbers of peptides. Advances in biotechnology are also enabling the development of new peptide-based materials, such as using genetic engineering to create peptides that can self-assemble into specific structures.

Researchers are also exploring new ways to interface peptides with biological systems, such as using peptides to target specific cells or tissues in the body or using peptides to create new types of biosensors or diagnostic tools. Advances in nanofabrication techniques are also allowing researchers to create complex peptide-based devices, such as microfluidic systems or bioelectronic devices. We strongly believe that peptide nanotechnology is an exciting and rapidly evolving field with the potential to revolutionize many areas of science and technology.

6.2 EMERGING TRENDS IN PEPTIDE NANOTECHNOLOGY

Peptide nanotechnology is a rapidly growing field that has the potential to revolutionize a wide range of applications, from medicine to materials science to electronics. As researchers continue to explore the properties and behavior of peptides, new trends are emerging (Figure 6.1) that are shaping the future of peptide nanotechnology.

One emerging trend in peptide nanotechnology is the use of peptides as building blocks for self-assembling materials. Peptides can spontaneously organize themselves into complex structures, making them an attractive option for the development of new materials. For example, peptide-based hydrogels can be used for tissue engineering and drug delivery,[1] while peptide-based nanofibers can be used for energy storage and electronic devices.[2]

Another emerging trend is the development of peptides as functional materials with specific properties. Researchers are exploring ways to design peptides with specific properties, such as catalytic activity, electrical conductivity, or magnetic properties. These functional peptides can be used for a wide range of applications, from sensors to electronic devices to energy storage.[2]

A third trend in peptide nanotechnology is the development of peptide-based therapeutics. Peptides can be used as therapeutic agents, targeting specific cells

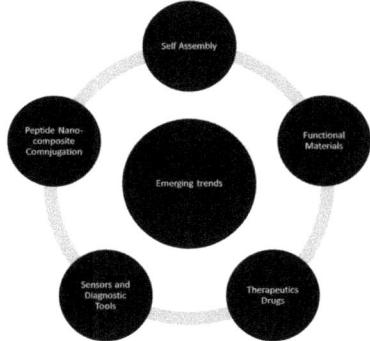

FIGURE 6.1 Schematic diagrams of peptides used in various forms and creating milestones by creating trends of such trades.

or tissues in the body with high specificity and efficiency. For example, peptide-based drugs have been developed for the treatment of cancer, diabetes, and other diseases. Peptide nanotechnology also offers new possibilities for drug delivery, allowing drugs to be delivered to specific locations in the body with greater precision and control.[3]

A fourth trend is the use of peptides as sensors and diagnostic tools. Peptides can be used to detect specific molecules with high sensitivity and specificity, making them ideal for use in diagnostic tests. For example, peptide-based biosensors have been developed that can detect biomarkers of disease, while peptide-based imaging agents can be used for diagnostic imaging.[4]

A fifth trend is the integration of peptides with nanotechnology. Peptides can be used to create nanoscale devices and structures, such as nanowires, nanotubes, and nanoparticles. These structures can be used for a wide range of applications, from electronics to drug delivery to environmental monitoring.[5]

To fully realize the potential of these emerging trends in peptide nanotechnology, several challenges must be overcome. One challenge is the design and synthesis of peptides themselves. Peptides are complex molecules that can have a wide range of properties, and designing peptides with specific properties can be difficult. In addition, synthesizing peptides can be a time-consuming and expensive process, making it difficult to scale up the production of peptide-based materials and devices.

Another challenge is the characterization of peptide-based materials and devices. Peptides can form complex structures that can be difficult to analyze using traditional characterization techniques, such as microscopy or spectroscopy. New techniques and tools will be needed to fully understand the properties and behavior of peptide-based materials and devices.

Peptides can interact with cells and tissues in complex ways, and understanding these interactions will be critical for the development of safe and effective peptide-based therapies. In addition, there is a need for understanding the environmental impact of peptide-based materials and devices, and how they can be safely disposed of or recycled.

Future directions and challenges in peptide nanotechnology

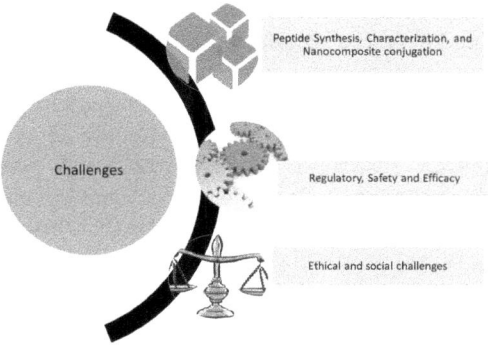

FIGURE 6.2 Various forms of challenges connected with peptide nanotechnology industry.

Emerging trends in peptide nanotechnology are opening up exciting possibilities for the future. Peptides have unique properties that make them attractive for a wide range of applications, and as researchers continue to explore the properties and behavior of peptides, new opportunities for innovation are likely to emerge. However, there are also significant challenges that must be overcome to fully realize the potential of peptide nanotechnology. By addressing these challenges as shown in Figure 6.2, researchers can continue to push the boundaries of what is possible with peptide-based materials and devices.

6.3 CHALLENGES IN PEPTIDE SYNTHESIS AND CHARACTERIZATION

Peptide synthesis and characterization are two critical aspects of peptide research. Peptides are complex molecules that play a crucial role in various fields, including medicine, biotechnology, and materials science. However, there are several challenges associated with peptide synthesis and characterization that must be overcome to develop effective peptide-based materials and therapies. Here are some key points that could be included in the challenges in peptide synthesis and characterization:

1. Complexity of peptide synthesis: The synthesis of peptides is a complex and challenging process that requires expertise in organic chemistry. Though peptides are made up of amino acids linked by peptide bonds, the synthesis process involves multiple steps that must be carefully controlled to ensure the correct sequence of amino acids. Additionally, the synthesis of longer peptides requires sophisticated strategies to prevent unwanted side reactions.[6]
2. Cost and time constraints: The synthesis of peptides can be expensive and time-consuming, especially for longer and more complex peptides. The cost of peptide synthesis can be a major barrier to research, particularly for smaller labs or academic researchers who may not have access

to the necessary resources. Improving the efficiency of peptide synthesis is critical to make it more accessible and affordable.

3. Purification and characterization: After synthesis, peptides must be purified and characterized to ensure their quality and efficacy. Purification can be challenging due to the complex mixture of products that are generated during synthesis. Characterization of peptides requires sophisticated techniques, such as mass spectrometry, nuclear magnetic resonance (NMR) spectroscopy, and circular dichroism (CD) spectroscopy, which can be costly and time-consuming.

4. Peptide conformation: The three-dimensional structure of a peptide is critical to its biological activity, and peptides can adopt a range of conformational states. However, determining the conformation of a peptide can be challenging, as it can be influenced by various factors, such as the solvent environment, pH, and temperature. Therefore, developing techniques that enable the characterization of peptide conformation is an important challenge.

5. Peptide aggregation: Peptides can aggregate into higher-order structures, such as fibrils, oligomers, and aggregates, which can affect their biological activity and lead to unwanted side effects. Aggregation can occur during synthesis or storage and can be influenced by a range of factors, such as temperature, pH, and solvent environment. Therefore, understanding the mechanisms of peptide aggregation and developing strategies to prevent it is a significant challenge.

6. Bioactivity of peptides: The biological activity of peptides is critical for their use in various applications, such as therapeutics, diagnostics, and materials science. However, the bioactivity of peptides can be affected by various factors, such as their conformation, aggregation state, and interactions with other molecules. Therefore, developing methods to measure and optimize the bioactivity of peptides is a crucial challenge.

7. Scale-up of peptide synthesis: The scale-up of peptide synthesis is essential for the production of larger quantities of peptides for use in various applications. However, scaling up the synthesis of peptides can be challenging due to issues such as reproducibility, purification, and yield. Developing strategies for scaling up peptide synthesis that are both efficient and cost-effective is an important challenge.[6]

Peptide synthesis and characterization are complex and challenging areas of research that require significant expertise and resources. Overcoming the challenges associated with peptide synthesis and characterization is critical for the development of effective peptide-based materials and therapies. Researchers must continue to develop innovative strategies and techniques to improve peptide synthesis and characterization and enable the full potential of peptides to be realized.

6.4 CHALLENGES IN PEPTIDE-BASED NANOMATERIALS

Peptide-based nanomaterials have emerged as a promising platform for the development of novel therapies, diagnostics, and materials science applications. Peptides are versatile molecules that offer numerous advantages, including high specificity, low toxicity, and biocompatibility. However, there are several challenges associated with the development and application of peptide-based nanomaterials. Here are some key points that could be included in the challenges in peptide-based nanomaterials:

1. Peptide synthesis: The synthesis of peptides is a complex and challenging process that requires expertise in organic chemistry. Peptides used for nanomaterials must be synthesized with high purity and in sufficient quantities to enable their use in various applications. Additionally, the synthesis of longer peptides or modified peptides can be more difficult and expensive. Therefore, improving the efficiency and cost-effectiveness of peptide synthesis is critical for the development of peptide-based nanomaterials.[7]
2. Stability and aggregation: Peptide-based nanomaterials can be prone to instability and aggregation, which can affect their performance and efficacy. Aggregation can occur due to various factors, including temperature, pH, and ionic strength.[8] Therefore, developing strategies to improve the stability and prevent aggregation of peptide-based nanomaterials is a significant challenge.
3. Bioactivity: The biological activity of peptide-based nanomaterials is critical for their use in various applications, including drug delivery and tissue engineering. However, the bioactivity of peptides can be affected by various factors, including their conformation, aggregation state, and interactions with other molecules. Therefore, developing methods to measure and optimize the bioactivity of peptide-based nanomaterials is a crucial challenge.
4. Targeting and specificity: Peptide-based nanomaterials can be engineered to target specific cells or tissues, which can improve their efficacy and reduce unwanted side effects. However, achieving high specificity and targeting can be challenging due to the complex environment of biological systems. Therefore, developing strategies to enhance the targeting and specificity of peptide-based nanomaterials is an important challenge.[9]
5. Toxicity: Peptide-based nanomaterials must be biocompatible and non-toxic to be used in biomedical applications. However, some peptides can be toxic or induce immune responses, which can limit their use. Therefore, developing methods to assess and reduce the toxicity of peptide-based nanomaterials is critical.[2]
6. Manufacturing and scale-up: The manufacturing and scale-up of peptide-based nanomaterials can be challenging due to issues such as reproducibility, quality control, and yield. Additionally, the manufacturing

process must be compatible with the intended application, such as drug delivery or tissue engineering. Therefore, developing efficient and cost-effective methods for manufacturing and scale-up of peptide-based nanomaterials is a significant challenge.
7. Regulatory approval: The regulatory approval of peptide-based nanomaterials can be challenging due to the complex nature of these materials and the potential for unwanted side effects. Therefore, developing strategies to ensure the safety and efficacy of peptide-based nanomaterials and obtaining regulatory approval is a crucial challenge.[10]

Nanomaterials with conjugated peptides offer numerous advantages for the development of novel therapies, diagnostics, and materials science applications. However, there are several challenges associated with the development and application of peptide-based nanomaterials that must be overcome to enable their full potential to be realized. Researchers must continue to develop innovative strategies and techniques to improve the stability, bioactivity, targeting, and manufacturing of peptide-based nanomaterials while ensuring their safety and regulatory approval.

6.5 REGULATORY CHALLENGES IN PEPTIDE-BASED THERAPEUTICS

Peptide-based therapeutics have shown great promise in the treatment of various diseases and disorders, such as cancer, diabetes, and autoimmune diseases. However, the development and approval of peptide-based therapeutics are subject to a range of regulatory challenges. Here are some key points that could be included in the regulatory challenges in peptide-based therapeutics:

1. Definition and classification: The definition and classification of peptide-based therapeutics are not straightforward, as they are often classified as both small molecules and biologics. Therefore, regulatory agencies must establish clear definitions and classifications for peptide-based therapeutics to ensure appropriate regulation and approval.
2. Manufacturing standards: The manufacturing of peptide-based therapeutics can be complex and challenging, as they are often produced using biological processes. Therefore, regulatory agencies must establish clear manufacturing standards and guidelines to ensure the consistency, purity, and quality of peptide-based therapeutics.[11]
3. Clinical trials: Clinical trials are a critical step in the development of peptide-based therapeutics, as they provide evidence of safety and efficacy. However, the design and conduct of clinical trials for peptide-based therapeutics can be challenging, as they require specialized expertise and knowledge. Therefore, regulatory agencies must establish clear guidelines and standards for the design and conduct of clinical trials for peptide-based therapeutics.

4. Safety and efficacy: The safety and efficacy of peptide-based therapeutics are critical for regulatory approval. However, assessing the safety and efficacy of peptide-based therapeutics can be challenging, as they may have complex mechanisms of action and interactions with the body. Therefore, regulatory agencies must establish clear guidelines and standards for assessing the safety and efficacy of peptide-based therapeutics.
5. Intellectual property: Intellectual property is a crucial aspect of the development and commercialization of peptide-based therapeutics. However, the patentability of peptide-based therapeutics can be challenging, as they are often derived from natural sources or are modifications of existing peptides. Therefore, regulatory agencies must establish clear guidelines and standards for the patentability of peptide-based therapeutics.
6. Post-market surveillance: Post-market surveillance is critical for monitoring the safety and efficacy of peptide-based therapeutics after they have been approved and are in use. However, post-market surveillance can be challenging for peptide-based therapeutics, as they may have complex mechanisms of action and interactions with the body. Therefore, regulatory agencies must establish clear guidelines and standards for post-market surveillance of peptide-based therapeutics.
7. Global harmonization: Peptide-based therapeutics are subject to regulation in multiple countries, and regulatory requirements can vary between countries. Therefore, global harmonization of regulatory requirements for peptide-based therapeutics is critical to facilitate the development and approval of these therapeutics and ensure patient safety.[11]

The development and approval of peptide-based therapeutics are subject to a range of regulatory challenges, including the definition and classification of these therapeutics, manufacturing standards, clinical trials, safety and efficacy assessments, intellectual property, post-market surveillance, and global harmonization of regulatory requirements. Regulatory agencies must establish clear guidelines and standards for these aspects of peptide-based therapeutics to ensure patient safety and enable the development and approval of these promising therapeutics.

6.6 ETHICAL AND SOCIAL CHALLENGES IN PEPTIDE NANOTECHNOLOGY

Peptide nanotechnology, which involves the design and application of nanoscale structures and materials composed of peptides (short chains of amino acids), has the potential to revolutionize various fields, including medicine, materials science, and electronics. However, like any emerging technology, it comes with ethical and social challenges that need to be carefully considered. Some of these challenges include:

1. Safety and toxicity: The use of peptide-based nanomaterials in medicine raises questions about their safety and potential toxicity. Ensuring

that these materials do not harm healthy cells or tissues is crucial while advances in peptide nanotechnology may lead to personalized medicine based on genetic information. This raises concerns about privacy, discrimination, and the misuse of sensitive genetic data.
2. Environmental impact: The production and disposal of peptide-based nanomaterials may have environmental consequences. Ensuring responsible manufacturing and waste management practices is essential.
3. Access and equity: Innovative medical treatments and technologies based on peptide nanotechnology must be accessible and affordable to all, regardless of socioeconomic status. Another factor is the global distribution of benefits and access to peptide nanotechnology should be equitable, avoiding further disparities in healthcare and technology between countries and populations.
4. Regulation and oversight: Developing appropriate regulatory frameworks for peptide nanotechnology to ensure safety and efficacy is challenging but necessary. While establishing standardized protocols and guidelines for the design, manufacturing, and testing of peptide nanomaterials is essential to ensure consistency and reliability.
5. Ethical use in research: Like many emerging technologies, peptide nanotechnology can be used for both beneficial and harmful purposes. Ethical considerations must guide research to prevent misuse.
6. Patents and ownership: Intellectual property rights and patents related to peptide nanotechnology can raise questions about access to knowledge and the concentration of power in the hands of a few.
7. Public awareness and engagement: Educating the public about the potential benefits and risks of peptide nanotechnology is crucial to promote informed decision-making. Involving the public in decision-making and governance related to peptide nanotechnology can help address concerns and ensure responsible development.
8. Cultural sensitivity: Peptide nanotechnology may intersect with cultural and ethical beliefs, particularly in the context of biotechnology and medicine. Respect for diverse perspectives is essential.
9. Biosecurity: There is a potential for the misuse of peptide nanotechnology in bioterrorism or other malicious activities. Adequate security measures and international cooperation are necessary to prevent such misuse.

Addressing these ethical and social challenges in peptide nanotechnology requires collaboration among scientists, policymakers, ethicists, and the public. An ethical and responsible approach to the development and deployment of these technologies is essential to maximize their benefits while minimizing potential harms.

6.7 FUTURE DIRECTIONS AND OPPORTUNITIES IN PEPTIDE NANOTECHNOLOGY

Peptide nanotechnology has emerged as an exciting and rapidly growing field with promising applications in biomedicine, materials science, and nanoelectronics.

Future directions and challenges in peptide nanotechnology   133

We will discuss some of the future directions and opportunities in peptide nanotechnology.

1. Multifunctional peptide nanomaterials: The development of multifunctional peptide nanomaterials that combine multiple properties, such as imaging, targeting, and therapeutic capabilities, is a promising direction in peptide nanotechnology. Multifunctional peptide nanomaterials could enable personalized medicine by providing targeted therapies with improved efficacy and reduced toxicity.
2. Peptide-based biosensors: The development of peptide-based biosensors that can detect specific molecules, such as proteins or small molecules, in real time is another promising direction in peptide nanotechnology. Peptide-based biosensors could be used for a range of applications, including disease diagnosis, drug discovery, and environmental monitoring.
3. Peptide-based drug delivery systems: The development of peptide-based drug delivery systems that can efficiently deliver therapeutic agents to specific tissues or cells is an exciting opportunity in peptide nanotechnology. Peptide-based drug delivery systems could improve the efficacy of existing drugs and enable the development of new therapies for diseases that are difficult to treat.
4. Self-assembling peptide nanomaterials: The development of self-assembling peptide nanomaterials that can form complex structures, such as nanotubes, nanofibers, and hydrogels, is an important direction in peptide nanotechnology. Self-assembling peptide nanomaterials could be used for tissue engineering, drug delivery, and regenerative medicine applications.
5. Peptide-based materials for energy applications: The development of peptide-based materials for energy applications, such as solar cells and batteries, is a promising opportunity in peptide nanotechnology. Peptide-based materials could offer advantages over traditional materials, such as improved stability and efficiency.
6. Peptide-based nanoelectronics: The development of peptide-based nanoelectronics that can be used in electronic devices, such as sensors, transistors, and memory devices, is an exciting direction in peptide nanotechnology. Peptide-based nanoelectronics could offer advantages over traditional materials, such as improved performance and biocompatibility.
7. Computational design of peptide nanomaterials: The development of computational methods for designing peptide nanomaterials with specific properties, such as self-assembly and stability, is an important opportunity in peptide nanotechnology. Computational design could enable the rapid and efficient development of new peptide nanomaterials with tailored properties for a range of applications.
8. Peptide-based vaccines: The development of peptide-based vaccines that can elicit specific immune responses is an important opportunity in peptide nanotechnology. Peptide-based vaccines could offer advantages over traditional vaccines, such as improved safety and specificity.

This is a rapidly growing field with promising applications in biomedicine, materials science, and nanoelectronics. The future directions and opportunities in peptide nanotechnology include the development of multifunctional peptide nanomaterials, peptide-based biosensors, peptide-based drug delivery systems, self-assembling peptide nanomaterials, peptide-based materials for energy applications, peptide-based nanoelectronics, computational design of peptide nanomaterials, and peptide-based vaccines. The continued advancement of peptide nanotechnology will enable the development of new and innovative solutions to some of the most challenging problems in science and medicine.

6.8 CONCLUSIONS AND FINAL THOUGHTS OF PEPTIDES IN NANOTECHNOLOGY

Peptide nanotechnology has emerged as an exciting field with promising applications in biomedicine, materials science, and nanoelectronics. Peptides, due to their unique physicochemical properties and biological functions, have been extensively explored as building blocks for the design and construction of novel nanomaterials. We have discussed various aspects of peptides in nanotechnology in this section, including synthesis and characterization challenges, regulatory challenges, emerging trends, and future directions.

One of the major challenges in peptide nanotechnology is the synthesis and characterization of peptide-based nanomaterials. The synthesis of peptides with high purity and yield is essential for the development of nanomaterials with predictable and reproducible properties. The use of automated peptide synthesis, solid-phase peptide synthesis, and recombinant DNA technology has greatly facilitated the synthesis of peptides with high purity and yield. However, the characterization of peptide-based nanomaterials is still challenging due to their complex structure and heterogeneity. Advanced analytical techniques, such as mass spectrometry, NMR spectroscopy, and X-ray crystallography, are required for the accurate characterization of peptide-based nanomaterials.

Regulatory challenges also exist in the development and commercialization of peptide-based therapeutics. Peptide-based therapeutics have unique properties that require specific regulatory considerations, such as the potential for immunogenicity, the difficulty in demonstrating bioequivalence, and the need for specialized manufacturing processes. Regulatory agencies, such as the Food and Drug Administration (FDA), have established guidelines for the development and approval of peptide-based therapeutics to ensure their safety and efficacy.

Despite the challenges, peptide nanotechnology has a promising future. Emerging trends in peptide nanotechnology include the development of multifunctional peptide nanomaterials, peptide-based biosensors, peptide-based drug delivery systems, self-assembling peptide nanomaterials, peptide-based materials for energy applications, peptide-based nanoelectronics, computational design of

Future directions and challenges in peptide nanotechnology 135

peptide nanomaterials, and peptide-based vaccines. These developments have the potential to revolutionize a range of fields, from healthcare to electronics.

One of the most promising areas of peptide nanotechnology is the development of peptide-based drug delivery systems. Peptide-based drug delivery systems have the potential to improve the efficacy of existing drugs and enable the development of new therapies for diseases that are difficult to treat. Peptide-based drug delivery systems can target specific tissues or cells, increase drug stability and bioavailability, and reduce toxicity. Several peptide-based drug delivery systems have already been approved for clinical use, and many more are in various stages of development.

Another exciting area of peptide nanotechnology is the development of self-assembling peptide nanomaterials. Self-assembling peptide nanomaterials have unique properties, such as biocompatibility, biodegradability, and the ability to form complex structures, that make them ideal for a range of applications, including tissue engineering, drug delivery, and regenerative medicine.

Peptide-based biosensors are another promising area of peptide nanotechnology. Peptide-based biosensors have the potential to detect specific molecules in real time, enabling the development of rapid and sensitive diagnostic tests for a range of diseases. Peptide-based biosensors can also be used for drug discovery and environmental monitoring.

Nevertheless, peptide nanotechnology is a rapidly growing field with promising applications in biomedicine, materials science, and nanoelectronics. While challenges exist, such as peptide synthesis and characterization, regulatory considerations, and safety concerns, the future of peptide nanotechnology is bright. The continued advancement of peptide nanotechnology will enable the development of new and innovative solutions to some of the most challenging problems in science and medicine. Peptide-based drug delivery systems, self-assembling peptide nanomaterials, and peptide-based biosensors are just a few examples of the exciting opportunities in peptides.

6.9 PRACTICAL QUESTIONS

1. What are some potential future applications of peptide nanotechnology, and how might they impact various industries?
2. What are the key challenges and obstacles that researchers face in advancing peptide nanotechnology for medical applications?
3. How can peptide-based nanomaterials be tailored for specific therapeutic purposes, and what are the challenges in achieving this level of precision?
4. What emerging techniques and methodologies hold promise for overcoming current limitations in peptide nanotechnology?
5. How can the scalability of peptide nanomaterial production be improved, and what role does sustainability play in the future of this field?

REFERENCES

1. Altunbas, A.; Pochan, D. J., Peptide-based and polypeptide-based hydrogels for drug delivery and tissue engineering. *Peptide-Based Materials* 2012, 310, 135–167.
2. Li, T.; Lu, X.-M.; Zhang, M.-R.; Hu, K.; Li, Z., Peptide-based nanomaterials: Self-assembly, properties and applications. *Bioactive Materials* 2022, 11, 268–282.
3. Sheehan, F.; Sementa, D.; Jain, A.; Kumar, M.; Tayarani-Najjaran, M.; Kroiss, D.; Ulijn, R. V., Peptide-based supramolecular systems chemistry. *Chemical Reviews* 2021, 121 (22), 13869–13914.
4. Karimzadeh, A.; Hasanzadeh, M.; Shadjou, N.; de la Guardia, M., Peptide based biosensors. *TrAC Trends in Analytical Chemistry* 2018, 107, 1–20.
5. Gao, X.; Matsui, H., Peptide-based nanotubes and their applications in bionanotechnology. *Advanced Materials* 2005, *17* (17), 2037–2050.
6. Bruckdorfer, T.; Marder, O.; Albericio, F., From production of peptides in milligram amounts for research to multi-tons quantities for drugs of the future. *Current Pharmaceutical Biotechnology* 2004, 5 (1), 29–43.
7. Yuan, L.; Liu, L., Peptide-based electrochemical biosensing. *Sensors and Actuators B: Chemical* 2021, *344*, 130232.
8. Wang, W.; Nema, S.; Teagarden, D., Protein aggregation—Pathways and influencing factors. *International Journal of Pharmaceutics* 2010, 390 (2), 89–99.
9. Dai, Q.; Bertleff-Zieschang, N.; Braunger, J. A.; Björnmalm, M.; Cortez-Jugo, C.; Caruso, F., Particle targeting in complex biological media. *Advanced Healthcare Materials* 2018, *7* (1), 1700575.
10. Varanko, A. K.; Chilkoti, A., Molecular and materials engineering for delivery of peptide drugs to treat type 2 diabetes. *Advanced Healthcare Materials* 2019, *8* (12), 1801509.
11. Rastogi, S.; Shukla, S.; Kalaivani, M.; Singh, G. N., Peptide-based therapeutics: Quality specifications, regulatory considerations, and prospects. *Drug Discovery Today* 2019, 24 (1), 148–162.

Index

advantages 2, 8, 9, 31, 33, 35, 36, 52, 54, 57, 58, 70, 72–75, 78, 95, 102–104, 111, 115, 116, 129, 130, 133
amino acids 30–36, 38, 39, 42, 43, 54, 75–77, 82, 83, 97, 102, 114, 115, 127, 131
amphiphilic peptides 54, 55
anticancer peptides (ACPs) 61, 84
antimicrobial peptides (AMPs) 5, 6, 55, 61, 72, 73, 84, 101
applications 1–4, 6–8, 10, 11, 15, 19, 23, 30, 33–35, 37, 38, 41, 44, 52–59, 61–65, 70, 72, 74–77, 79–83, 85, 95–97, 99, 101–104, 106, 111, 112, 124–135

bacteria 6, 18, 72, 73, 84, 101, 109, 114
biocompatibility of peptides 1, 3, 5, 8, 10, 11, 53, 55–58, 64, 70, 71, 73, 83, 103, 104, 129, 133, 135
biological synthesis 15, 31, 34, 42, 109, 129
biosensors 2–4, 10–11, 52–56, 58, 61, 95–101, 125, 126, 133–135
blood brain barrier (BBB) 80, 96, 110
body 8, 39, 55, 63, 76, 84, 85, 96, 107, 109, 110, 112, 124–126, 131

cancer cells 3, 72, 74, 76, 81, 84, 96, 107, 108, 110–117
cancer therapy 4, 10, 74, 84, 96, 111
carbon 2, 4, 5, 23, 27, 41, 57, 59, 71, 100
cell-penetrating peptides (CPPs) 77
challenges 8, 9, 11, 19, 23, 27, 28, 30, 33, 36, 37, 83–87, 111, 117, 124–132, 134, 135
characterization of peptides 1, 2, 9, 11, 15, 19, 32, 36–43, 63, 124, 126–128, 134, 135
chemical synthesis of peptides 15, 18, 19
chemotherapy 111, 112, 116
classification of peptides 6, 53, 75, 130
CPP-mediated 76–79

damage 6, 73, 81, 82, 114
development 2–8, 10, 11, 19, 20, 28, 31, 33–35, 37–43, 54, 60, 65, 71–75, 77, 79, 81, 84, 85, 99–102, 104–106, 111–114, 116, 117, 124–126, 128–135
disease diagnosis 11, 99–101, 107–109, 111, 133
drug delivery systems 3, 10, 11, 74, 75, 77, 80, 82, 86, 87, 133–135
dye 6, 56, 58, 64, 107, 110

employed 2, 4, 19, 23, 31, 41, 44, 62, 63, 74, 79, 80, 82, 86, 87, 96, 101, 104, 115
engineering 1–11, 34, 35, 38, 44, 52–55, 57, 58, 62–64, 82, 96, 101–106, 125, 129, 130, 133, 135
environmental monitoring 97, 99–101, 126, 133, 135
ethical challengers 131, 132

factors 3, 33, 36, 52, 54, 55, 57–59, 84, 86, 102, 128–129
functional 6–8, 11, 16, 21, 23–25, 27–29, 32, 34–36, 40, 42, 59, 60, 63, 71, 97, 102, 104, 106, 125
future directions 124, 132–135

healthy 59, 71, 74, 76, 80–84, 86, 102, 116, 117, 132
high-performance liquid chromatography (HPLC) 9, 15, 19, 28, 39, 40, 42
historical background 4, 34
hybrid peptide synthesis 34–38, 62, 76, 87, 104, 107
hydrogels 5, 6, 38, 56, 63–65, 75, 76, 103–106, 124, 125, 133

identification 15, 42, 43, 81, 107, 116
imaging agents 6, 10, 11, 55, 56, 58, 64, 79, 86, 107–109, 112, 126
imaging and diagnostics 10, 106
immune 8, 10, 38, 74, 75, 81, 85, 111–116, 129, 133
inhibitors 72, 96, 113, 115

liposomes 4, 70–72, 75, 76, 81

mass spectrometry for peptide characterization 2, 9, 15, 19, 40–43, 128, 134
materials 2, 4–8, 11, 23, 30, 32, 38–43, 53, 55–59, 62–64, 70, 82, 83, 95, 97, 102, 103, 124–135
mechanisms 17, 54, 78, 80, 81, 84, 94, 100, 103, 117, 128, 131
microscopy 40, 62, 63, 110, 111, 124–126

nanocomposites 62
nanoparticles 2–6, 10, 52, 55, 70–75, 81, 83, 96, 97, 101, 107, 112, 116, 126

nanotechnology 1–12, 53, 63, 86, 124–127, 131–135
nanotubes and nanorods 57–59, 61
NMR spectroscopy 9, 15, 19, 40–43, 128, 134
non-ribosomal peptide synthesis 17, 18

optimization 28, 33, 36, 37, 83, 111–113

peptide amphiphilic 54
peptide characterization methods 9, 15, 40–43
peptide nucleic acids (PNAs) 5, 79, 134
peptide self-assembly 43, 53, 54, 106
peptide-based 1–11, 38–40, 43, 52, 55–57, 62–65, 70–76, 85, 86, 95–116, 124–135
properties of peptides 2, 7, 40, 54, 99
prospects of peptides-based 11, 64, 85, 86
purification and characterization 32, 36–40, 128
purification of peptides 33, 38, 39, 42
quantum dots 79

rapid 19, 28, 40, 43, 73, 74, 114, 133, 135
regulatory challenges 130, 131, 134
ribosomal synthesis of peptides 17, 18

scaffolds 52, 62, 102, 103, 106, 108
self-assembling peptides (SAPs) 5, 6, 52–55, 58–60, 62, 105, 106, 133

solid-phase peptide synthesis (SPPS) 1, 18–20, 30, 35, 134
spectroscopy 9, 15, 19, 40–43, 62, 63, 124, 126, 128, 134
stimuli-responsive peptides 11, 82, 83, 87
substance 37, 71, 77, 103
synthesis of peptides 15, 17–20, 28, 29, 36, 37, 124, 126–129, 134

targeted drug delivery 9, 37, 59, 60, 62, 71, 79–81, 125, 126, 128, 130, 134
techniques 2–4, 6, 8–10, 15, 18, 19, 28, 29, 32, 33, 38–41, 43, 55, 56, 58, 61–63, 80, 81, 86, 105, 108–111, 124–126, 128, 130, 134–135
tissue engineering 1–11, 38, 52–55, 57, 58, 62–64, 96, 101–106, 124, 125, 129, 130, 133, 135

vaccines 10, 76, 78, 112–116, 133–135
variety of application/industry/solution 3, 4, 7–9, 11, 19, 30, 38, 40, 42, 52, 53, 59–61, 64, 70, 71, 74, 77–82, 97, 101, 105, 107, 111
vectors 103

water 19, 23, 56, 59, 61, 64, 68, 76, 82, 99, 100, 103, 105

X-ray crystallography 2, 41, 134
XLAsp-P2 55

For Product Safety Concerns and Information please contact our EU
representative GPSR@taylorandfrancis.com
Taylor & Francis Verlag GmbH, Kaufingerstraße 24, 80331 München, Germany

www.ingramcontent.com/pod-product-compliance
Ingram Content Group UK Ltd.
Pitfield, Milton Keynes, MK11 3LW, UK
UKHW041130300825
462417UK00007B/78